Yoga complete for Weight loss

Roger Barton

Contents

Introduction

The Yogic Approach

In today's hectic and overstuffed culture, it may be difficult to make good food choices and stick to a regular exercise routine. It requires making significant, well-considered adjustments to one's lifestyle and trying out new combinations of one's distinct but complementary talents in the fields of diet, physical activity, psychology, and spirituality.

The Effect Will Last Forever

There are no quick fixes that will bring about lasting improvement. The willingness to alter one's way of life for the better and to face and conquer negative habits is crucial. Be prepared to let go of any preconceived notions you may have about healthy eating and activity, as well as any emotional walls you may have created around food. There is currently no simple answer to the problem of obesity. Body, mind, and spirit are all impacted by eating disorders. Consequently, it is necessary to adopt a comprehensive approach that considers these factors.

The coming together of faith and reason (rational)

Develop your faith to get some perspective. With this level of insight, you'll be less tempted by quick solutions and more committed to decisions with lasting effects on your life. If we have a clear sense of why we're here, it may encourage us to make healthier food and activity decisions. One another's affection and respect will serve as a guiding force in your development into responsible, self-reliant adults. Your newfound independence will allow you to put the long-term benefits of a balanced diet ahead of the short-term pleasure of junk food. To have access to your true wealth — a healthy body upon which to construct a meaningful life — you must take responsibility for your health and stop relying on others to keep you alive and well. A newfound glow of joy illuminates everything of existence.

Yoga (Body)

"Yoga" is a spiritual practise for weight loss that literally means "union" in Sanskrit. Yoga, if practised frequently, may be useful in this regard, but perhaps not in the manner one first expects. Yoga aids fitness by encouraging a mental change that lays the way for permanent lifestyle modifications, so you may get the health benefits of a leaner, more flexible body without tracking calories or lifting weights. Mind and body peace that doesn't need effort to maintain may be achieved via regular practise of Yoga's eight limbs. With such confidence, you'll be able to see things more clearly, make more informed decisions, and deal with any challenge with ease.

Physical yoga has gained popularity across the globe, and some individuals do include it into their workouts, but the yoga tradition as a whole provides a comprehensive approach to self-improvement. Yoga is beneficial for your mind and soul as well as your body. It helps us reach our full potential by balancing our physical, mental, and spiritual selves. When yoga is practised in tandem with Ayurveda, an ancient Indian medicinal tradition, healing becomes both simpler and more potent. Ayurveda and Yoga are complementary healing practises that include the whole individual, not only the physical or mental symptoms. It has been shown that consistent yoga practise improves not only physical health but also mental and emotional well-being. Yoga has the potential to alter one's perspective on health, fitness, and nutrition. Because of everything you've learned about respect and love for your body in yoga, you feel more inclined to eat whole, natural meals rather than manufactured junk food. The best way to lose weight is to modify your thinking rather than blindly adhere to a new diet plan.

Traditional approaches to weight reduction just target the outward signs (body fat) and do not deal with the underlying causes of the issue (an imbalance manifested in a number of different ways, including emotional problems, unhealthy behaviours, and nutritional inadequacies). A yogi's primary objective is not caloric expenditure like that of an ordinary gym-goer. Aerobic exercise aids in weight loss since it increases metabolism and decreases appetite. The question is whether or not it will really make you feel better on the inside, and whether or not that improvement in mood will translate into long-term success with your weight reduction efforts. Calorie counting is not an useful weight reduction approach since it is tedious and stressful to keep track of one's food intake on a regular basis.

Yoga's benefits extend well beyond just weight loss, thanks to the discipline and awareness it fosters in its practitioners. Practicing yoga will provide you a powerful incentive to enhance the quality of the food you feed your body. Someone's likes and dislikes of certain foods may change as they become older and their taste receptors develop. People may be motivated to eat better, practise mindfulness, and put themselves first if this occurs. It's conceivable that committing to a regular yoga practise can inspire you to make positive changes to the way you eat and live. Use any combination of these strategies if you really want to shed pounds and keep them off. When you've spent an exhausting hour at the gym, doing some yoga is a terrific way to unwind and may help you deal with any underlying emotional problems that might be causing your weight gain. Consistent yoga practise has been linked to positive health and metabolic effects, as well as increased calm and control of one's emotional state. Maintaining a healthy weight is one of the many obstacles in life that requires a level head and self-discipline.

Chapter: 1

Tangible and Intangible Yoga Influences

A regular yoga practise may be one of the best and healthiest strategies to keep the pounds off. In addition to increasing satiety and speeding up your metabolism, it also improves your mood, self-esteem, and, most significantly, your appreciation for the sacredness of your own being. The moral and spiritual basis of yoga might give you the will to overcome an enemy as formidable as the incessant, even overpowering, want to eat.

For you, the most important question is whether or not yoga can help you lose weight. One of the six basic benefits of yoga is a reduction in body weight.

1: First, it aids in sating your hunger pangs. Yoga has been demonstrated to have real, measurable physiological impacts on the body's hunger centre, and it also has the additional benefit of altering one's outlook on themselves. You've gained more mobility, flexibility, and readiness. As a result, many individuals will heave a sigh of relief. After experiencing and appreciating it, and then comparing how you feel before and after a substantial meal, you can come to realise that there are other types of pleasure than eating. It's the kind of feeling that remains with you for years.

2: This phenomena directly causes people to change their eating habits. Fewer fried foods, less sugar, fewer processed foods, and more vegetables are what the "lifestyle change advocates" over the last 30 years have recommended. The books **Forks Over Knives** by **Gene Stone** and **The Acid Watcher Diet** by **Dr. Jonathan Aviv** are quite similar to one another. The subtle benefits of yoga inspire the same conduct as advocated by these authorities, who are often referred to as gurus. Vegetables are a crucial element of a yogi's diet.

PGC-1alpha (more on that intriguing chemical, along with mitochondria and telomeres, later) and the protection of antidiabetic pathways have been established in recent studies on a wide range of edible plants. Those who are healthier and live longer have a preference for a diet high in colourful, non-grilled fruits and vegetables.

3: Increases metabolic rate by boosting mitochondrial synthesis and activity. The benefits of PGC-1alpha, the body's stimulant for larger and more productive mitochondria, have never been quantified; however, the extraordinary bodies, high levels of fitness, and peak performance of the vast majority of dedicated yogis speak volumes. This emphasises the significance of diverting glucose away from fatty tissue storage and toward use in energy production.

4: You can think of four main ways in which it will be useful. Weight Watchers may have found success because they take a comprehensive approach to dieting by providing both nutritional guidance and social support. A few years ago, they rebranded themselves from a diet company to one that uses group meetings to promote a new lifestyle and a line of low-calorie meals. One of the company's open secrets for the future appears to be the use of peer-group elements as a way of advertising this way of life. People who practise yoga often socialise with those who have similar interests. There is a group dynamic similar to that of Weight Watchers, but nobody is required to attend on a weekly basis and members are not required to weigh in. The benefits to one's overall health, not just one's weight, are highlighted, as are the small or nonexistent costs involved when compared to the previous scarcity of goods available.

5: The practise of yoga seems to be the bedrock of self-discipline, which is the bedrock of successful weight management. Self-discipline can be thought of as the disposition to recognise and follow one's own superior judgement. Success in reaching your goals depends on your level of self-control. Doing the opposite of what you naturally want to do is a virtue in and of itself. To follow through on your plans, you must be internally committed to doing so. Just such a focused determination to succeed can be fostered through the practise of yoga. **Asana** (or "yoga postures") practise has become so commonplace in Western culture that it often surprises onlookers. Until now, I've never met anyone who could say, "I've always been consistent with everything I've done." Like those old Honda commercials, yoga has a positive feedback loop that keeps drawing new practitioners.

6: Regular yoga practise creates and sustains an inner confidence, a quiet "Yes I can" that permeates one's entire being. Self-discipline and an optimistic outlook are the cornerstones of willpower. 1

Beyond the physical benefits of yoga, there are many more reasons to take up the practise if you want to lose weight. From what we can tell, yoga was developed as a means of personal development, a means of breaking free of the constraints of daily life. All over the world, people from different cultures have been moved by the practice's hypnotic allure and calming effect. There has been a phantom pendulum swing in yoga's popularity from contemplation of **Nirvana** and **eternal bliss** to more mundane concerns. In the last two decades, many people have considered yoga's potential to aid in the resolution of global problems. Clinical trials have shown efficacy for a variety of diseases. Even though it hasn't been proven, I believe it could help bring about world peace.

It's safe to say that the ancient yogis' ways of life were as varied as their practises. Like the vast majority of modern yoga practitioners, many of these individuals had active lives outside of their yoga practise, including families, careers, and other pursuits. Still others were spiritual advisors, teachers, or doctors who worked in the mansions of the wealthy but lived in communities that were intentionally isolated from the rest of society. The spiritual practises of meditation and mindfulness remain at the forefront, and yoga is increasingly being used as a medical treatment for everything from the side effects of chemotherapy on cancer patients to the age-old issues of not getting enough sleep and being overweight.

Like the beauty in some works of Japanese art that lie in the blank spaces between the lines, the spiritual dimension of the process is implicit. With these "higher" associations in mind, yoga can be an even more effective tool in the sometimes simple, sometimes difficult process of losing weight.

Yes, it is possible to do so. Please have faith. The well-documented health benefits of yoga may give you the confidence you need to adopt this ancient practise. Being overweight is linked to numerous health issues, some of which can be fatal; yoga has the potential to treat or even reverse many of these conditions. I'll also give pointers on how to modify yoga poses for people with extra weight and the health issues that often come along with it.

Chapter: 2

Benefits for Conditions Related to Overweight

Medical:

1: HYPERTENSION (HIGH BLOOD PRESSURE):

Herbert Benson's "relaxation reaction" is simultaneously one of the most shocking and logical conclusions regarding yoga. The blood pressure of those with hypertension may drop by 10 to 20 points with frequent practise of yoga-based meditation. Although first met with scepticism from the medical world, Dr. Benson's groundbreaking study has been replicated, accepted, and adopted time and time again in the more than 40 years since its publication.

Emergence of Diabetic Illness

2: Diabetes:

It may be greatly improved or even cured by adhering to the dietary restrictions associated with yoga, which often include meditation and physical postures. This study was conducted in India and was headed by Dr. Kim Innes.

3: Heart Attack,

Numerous studies have shown that the lifestyle modifications associated with yoga have the ability to considerably increase the working width of the coronary arteries and, in turn, blood flow to the heart. Several reputable scientists are beginning to give yoga more consideration because of the potential benefits it may have in improving health and wellbeing via changes in diet and exercise.

4: ASTHMA

Yogis have practised **pranayama**, or yogic **breathing practises**, for thousands of years, and many people believe it may help with asthma. In order to control his asthma, B.K.S. **Iyengar**, one of the world's most renowned yoga teachers, reportedly began practising yoga at a young age. Although several studies have shown that yoga has no effect on lung function in people with asthma, some researchers still believe that it may help asthma sufferers. Four was the tension level.

5: Stress

In the same laboratory where Walter B. Cannon discovered the famous "**fight or flight**" response to perceived danger in the 1920s, Harvard psychiatry professor Herbert Benson, MD, developed the "rest and digest" reaction to meditation. When faced with danger, however, many people find that their anxiety and tension levels rise, whereas meditation has the opposite impact. Even in places where teenage hypertension is relatively uncommon, Benson's findings have been corroborated.

6: Lower Back Pain

Back discomfort is a typical reason people start doing yoga. Due to the wide variety of potential reasons, a thorough assessment of the individual's problem is necessary before commencing yoga for the temporary relief or long-term therapy of back pain. Treatment for back pain or sciatica often begins with pain medication. A huge difference might be made if these promising findings were applicable to other conditions such as lumbar disc herniation and spinal stenosis. The usefulness and adaptability of yoga cannot be denied.

7: Metastatic Cancer

However, yoga, in particular, has been shown to have a positive influence on the quality of life of cancer patients and survivors by reducing stress and anxiety. In addition to the more apparent physical benefits of greater mobility, strength, and posture, there are also positive effects on mental health, socialisation, and depression reduction. The seven s stand for osteoporosis.

8: Osteoporosis

From my 15 years of study, I have derived a 12-minute yoga programme for patients with osteopenia and osteoporosis, as well as healthy people who don't want either ailment. Previous research has shown that yoga may increase bone mineral density, an effect that seems to last into old age.

9: Arthritis

Seven Arthritis Yoga may help arthritis because it stretches the muscles, which increases flexibility at the endpoints of motion that are often limited by arthritis. Inconclusive evidence suggests that yoga may help reduce the discomfort associated with rheumatic diseases like rheumatoid arthritis, but this is just a hypothesis. The ninth swing in temperament.

10: Depression

Studies utilising various types of yoga for depression have shown encouraging outcomes, leading to the development of a number of yoga-based therapies ranging from Tantric meditation to the more classic hatha yoga headstand.

Yoga might be a great mood-booster if you're feeling down in the dumps.

11: SCOLIOSIS

Childhood scoliosis increased as the frequency of polio and cerebral palsy declined. The word "idiopathic" is used when doctors have no idea what's causing a certain ailment. By comparison of pre-and post-treatment x-rays, yoga has been found to be effective for both the degenerative type of adult scoliosis and adolescent idiopathic scoliosis.

12: Rotator Cuff Syndrome

It's not uncommon to suffer from rotator cuff syndrome or an actual rotator cuff injury.

Shoulder discomfort and limited arm mobility are symptoms of rotator cuff dysfunction. There is some evidence that regular yoga practise might alleviate these issues.

13: Anxiety

The National Institutes of Health is using this strategy to investigate pain. Multiple, high-quality studies have shown that different yoga practises are helpful in reducing anxiety.Yoga, like medicine, might provide both short-and long-term benefits for depression.

14: Career-Related Stress Disorder (PTSD)

Even if their injuries are too severe for even the most advanced medical technology to treat, they may benefit greatly from the meditative "parallel play" of yoga. As a result of its success in treating PTSD, yoga is now offered in more than **125 VA** hospitals and clinics (PTSD).

Yoga has several potential benefits, including helping with weight loss.

So far, we've examined the therapeutic advantages of yoga, which may be categorised into a broad range of treatments for a wide range of conditions. However, what about actual people now? People who are able to practise yoga may gain advantages beyond the sphere of physical wellness. While being overweight increases one's risk of several health problems, it is not a disease in and of itself.

1: MEMORY

Multiple scientific studies and an almost infinite number of anecdotal accounts have shown that yoga improves both working and long-term memory. Consistent users attribute half of the benefits to the cognitive enhancement and the other half to the psychological benefits of increased focus and calm.

2: Posture

Yoga's attention to the spine has been shown to have a direct, positive effect on the body's posture. Damage is done to the person's health, happiness, and sense of self-worth.

3: BALANCE

The issue lies in attempting to pin down the essence of balance in a definition. Nouns may disappear first when a balance starts to shift. This kind of disproportion may sometimes manifest itself even while the person is at rest. The verb form refers not just to the physical skill shown by gymnasts and other sports, but also to the act of coming back to one's own centre after being knocked off balance. Yoga has been demonstrated to improve a wide variety of physical abilities, not only balance and mobility.

4: Strength and range of motion:

In order to get the benefits of yoga, such as improved strength and flexibility, it is necessary to maintain challenging poses for extended periods of time.

Age 19 will give you a deeper understanding of these necessities for maintaining your health.

5: FACTUAL CAPABILITY

Recent studies demonstrate that yoga may improve patients' overall capacity to undertake a range of activities, adding support to the idea that it might help in the recovery of medical diseases like stroke.

6: Pregnancy

A baby's development is well underway by the 20th week of pregnancy.

Some research has connected prenatal yoga to an easier labour and delivery.

7: General Coordination

State-of-the-art-electrophysiological-research suggests that even eight weeks of yoga practice may have a major impact on performance among young Indians.

8: Thickened cortical layers five in the brain

It seems that the most highly developed of the brain's six cortical layers responds most strongly to yoga. Despite the fact that each layer performs a unique job, the loss of layers has been linked to cognitive impairment. Yoga practise has been shown to slow the rate of brain atrophy in the elderly.

Neuropsychological assessments revealed that after just eight weeks of yoga, participants had considerable improvements in their sense of self and confidence.

9: Self Esteem

For a society plagued by addiction and low self-esteem, this may be yoga's greatest strength.

Exercises that help you change course and permanently close the fat door in your face.

10: Weight Loss

Even though it is not the main focus of the book, I decided to include it here since it is one of the many advantages of yoga. I'm aware that there are many who disagree, but I still count this as one of yoga's positive effects. From my perspective, yoga has potential benefits for weight management.

Chapter: 3

Do You Really Need to Lose Weight?

At this point, you may be persuaded that yoga is effective enough to aid in weight loss. But the question may come up, as it does with so many delays and sidesteps in life: Is there a need for this? Surely there must be a wide variety of views on what constitutes the "ideal" weight in the globe. Is there such such thing as an ideal weight? It may be like wearing a suit or a dress, perhaps. Because of the wide variety of possible contexts and individual preferences, there is no "right" approach.

The human body is too varied for a "**one size fits all**" approach. The somatotyping method developed by 1940s psychologist William Herbert Sheldon was an early effort to acknowledge this. He classified human bodies into three groups:

1: Ectomorph (thin, delicate, rapid metabolism, trouble gaining weight)

2: .Mesomorph (large-boned and well-muscled; tough and athletic; "rectangular form").

3: Endomorph (round shape, fatty tissue, slow metabolism, trouble losing weight)

Named after the three primary tissues present in the embryonic development process, ectoderm (skin and nervous system), mesoderm (muscle and bone), and endoderm (gut and blood vessels) (digestive system). Sheldon even attempted to use this approach to categorise individuals according to their emotional and behavioural tendencies, but it backfired. Some folks, especially during the holiday season, appeared to switch personalities. The results of the system were inconclusive in the end.

The body mass index (BMI) scale was developed by Belgian mathematician **Lambert Adolphe Jacques Quetelet** in the early nineteenth century to apply mathematical approaches to the life sciences; it was accepted in the United States in 1998. The logic behind this was that unlike weeds, human beings do not gain mass according to their height (a linear measure), nor do they gain mass like pumpkins by increasing their spherical radius (which would entail the cube root of their size). Human development occurs between these two extremes. Weight (in kilos) divided by height (**in square metres**) gives the **Quetelet's index**.

The BMI is a broad instrument that functions best when used to big populations. Application to specific people is cautioned, but we may use the rules it provides very effectively moving forward. One is considered underweight if their BMI is less than 18, healthy weight is between **18** and **25**, overweight is **25** to **29.9**, and obese is **30** or above on the scale. So, if you're **5** feet, **4** inches tall and weigh **146** pounds, you're overweight. The BMI cutoff for obesity is **175**. If you are **6** feet and **1** inch tall, you are considered overweight if your weight is **190**, and obese if it is **228**. It's instructive to have a look at where you fall on this spectrum.

Let's face it, there are certain restrictions with this setup. Not all sexes, not all ages, and not all races can be described by a single formula. The integumentary system, which includes our skin and hair, is the body's biggest organ and is naturally thicker in women than in males. Some racial and ethnic groups have different metabolic rates than others. These variations are not very big, but they have been confirmed by rigorous research.

As a result, Professor David Fah of Geneva, Switzerland, has collaborated on the development of the Smart Body Mass Index (SBMI). The "smart" BMI doesn't wow me with its brainpower. It's still rather indifferent to the many ways in which people are unique, and its cutoff points are much too generous. Shouldn't a smart system take into account the fact that conditions like high blood pressure, arthritis, and diabetes might have a significant impact on your ideal body mass index?

To prepare for the possibility of disease or digestive dysfunction as we age, proponents of the Smart Body Mass Index recommend that we put on weight (one proposal is a pound every year over the age of 60). Aside from those who are already overweight, I agree it is sound advice. Even in theory, this system has flaws, since it encourages putting on weight as you get older to increase your chances of survival in dangerous situations, but it also puts a lot of strain on your body's nonfat tissues (such as your internal organs, blood, tendons, ligaments, nerves, and muscles). Only muscle mass can be altered by us. According to Smart BMI, increasing muscle mass is a crucial part of maintaining a healthy weight in old age. Muscle bulk increases energy consumption even while resting, therefore this may have the

unintended consequence of depleting older people's energy stores.
Neither of these methods is foolproof, but based on my years of practise as a doctor, I would recommend using the BMI as a starting point and then tailoring an individual's optimum weight to their own health needs.
There does not seem to be a single, agreed-upon technique to determine which criteria to utilise in determining whether or not you are excessively overweight or dangerously underweight. As such, I advocate utilising the BMI with certain caveats. In order to get an accurate BMI reading if you suffer from hypertension or diabetes, you should subtract **5–7** percent from your calculated weight in order to get a more accurate reading; if you have a tendency toward anorexia or a chronic digestive condition, you should add to your calculated weight in order to get an accurate reading. Given our existing limitations, I believe this to be the most helpful and convenient method for determining your precise weight right now.

These methods seem to be the most cutting-edge in medicine today for determining whether you should maintain your current weight, lose weight, or gain weight as you get older, and if so, by how much. They also provide information about whether or not the weight change is medically significant, which may be a very inspiring factor. It is clear that the medical benefits of losing weight go well beyond what is included in these recommendations. The effectiveness of anticancer treatments, heart disease, and lung disease are all negatively impacted by obesity. You may use these things to help you stick to your decision. That is something that we shall discuss later. It's time to look at the other assessments that answer the first, most important question: Do you need to reduce weight?

TAKEN ON YOUR OWN TERMS

Medical ramifications of being overweight are awful things that may happen, but we are often too preoccupied to do something about it. In such scenario, you may want to consider certain non-objective factors. It's not necessary to write yourself a note letting you know if you're feeling uneasy since you already know.

Being "**at ease in one's own skin**" is a good starting point. Are you pushed forward by your belly as you go in or out of the shower? Is it because you have large thighs that you have to sit with your legs crossed in the backseat of your car? Does your size limit or prevent you from engaging in certain intimate positions? You can know these things while wearing just your birthday suit.

Can you go up one flight of stairs without feeling out of breath? Think well of yourself when you look in the mirror? Is your belly so big that it hurts your back when you lift heavy loads?

Plus, forget about your skin. How about apparel? If your stomach bulges through the space between the button and the buttonhole, or if your feet haven't altered much in the last fifteen years yet your shoes are too tight, you may experience some discomfort.

CONTESTANTS IN THE YOGA

Yoga may help you find out whether you're having problems with your balance, agility, or general fitness (which includes strength) since it's a practise that emphasises relaxation, flexibility, and equilibrium. First, let's talk about how being overweight might hinder your equilibrium, which becomes more and more important as you get older.

Vriksasan*a*

The Trunk of the Tree (a variation)

The benefits and mechanism of action are as follows: as this position requires a good deal of balance, it helps those who already have good balance and reveals those who do not to try it. This modification of the traditional position is safe for people who might otherwise struggle with it, while yet being rigorous enough to reveal imbalances in a person's equilibrium.

Warning: If you have plantar fasciitis, a sprained ankle, or poor balance, you shouldn't do this position. When one foot hurts (from plantar fasciitis or a damaged ankle, for example), the other can take the load.

CONTOURING FOR THE PERFECT STANCE

THE POSE

1: With your back against a wall and the chair to your right, turn the chair such that its side is braced against the wall and facing you.

2: Spread your toes and stand with your feet about hip-width apart. Put all of your weight onto your left foot by pressing down on the ball and heel. Moderately contract your left quads and hamstrings to tighten up your whole leg. Simply tucking in the buttocks and bringing the lower pelvis forward can give you a little hip extension. Follow these steps and you should see a decrease in your lumbar curvature.
3: Put your pelvis over your feet in a straight line. Raise your right foot and rest it, toes pointing away from you, on the chair's seat.
4: Keep your pelvis looking forward as you gently and deliberately move your right bent knee and leg out to the side (ideally at ninety degrees to the left foot).
5: Look at anything fifteen to twenty feet away and at eye level.
6: Take a deep breath in while you optionally lift both arms over your head, palms facing each other, with the biceps as far behind the ears as possible without causing your head to jut forward. Just be sure to breathe all the air into your lungs.
Stretch from your left ankle to your head and then out to your thumbs and fingers.
7: Bring your shoulder blades together behind you. Stomach forward till you can stand without the wall. Lengthen your limbs toward the clouds.
8: Now, gently and slowly, remove your right foot from under the seat. Put your foot back down if you feel yourself leaning forward.

9: Now do it again, this time with your left foot on the chair.

A good goal would be to maintain this posture for fifteen seconds. If you can't, you probably need to work on your balance. Just though you can maintain the stance for a few seconds is no indication that you don't need to reduce weight, but the opposite is also true. Even if you aren't overweight, if you have a tendency to lose your balance in less than fifteen seconds, you should work to improve it. If your results indicate that your balance is substantially poorer than you recall it being in the past, this is extremely crucial. When it comes to restoring equilibrium, Yoga is equally as effective as it is in spotting its absence. As your stability grows, you may take this posture farther.

This stance, along with others like it, will be discussed in much more depth later on. Simply making note of the outcomes and moving on to determine whether your mobility is impaired is adequate at this stage. You'll need to get on the floor for this one.

Marichyasana I.
Spin while seated (variation)

The ribs prevent the thoracic spine from twisting excessively, and the forward and backward motion of the lumbar vertebral facets similarly limits rotation. This means that the **T12-L1** area of the spine is responsible for the vast majority of the twisting motion. Yet the twist causes pressure to be maintained in the lumbar and thoracic spines. This means the position is beneficial for osteoporosis sufferers as well. It's a great way to strengthen your bones.

If you have a herniated disc then you shouldn't twist in this direction. Be easy on yourself if you suffer from facet arthritis or facet syndrome; the alternative postures suggested below may serve as more reliable control groups. After having surgery on your hips or lower back, or having had a hip replaced from the rear, this stance should be avoided.

CONTOURING FOR THE PERFECT STANCE

The pose

1: Sit on a rug or a mat with your legs spread apart.

2: To straighten your back, press your hands into the floor beside you.

3: With your right knee bent, put your right foot on the mat next to your left thigh's thickest region. Set your left foot firmly on the ground and extend your leg all the way through the sole of your foot to position.

4: Keeping the big toe side of your foot upright, extend it forward.

5: With your next breath, straighten your back and twist to the right.

6: Position your left upper arm outside your right knee. To avoid rounding your back, slide it forward to contact the outside of the folded knee as far up on the arm as feasible. You may choose to fully extend your arm and hold it there if you want.

7: Position your left upper arm or armpit on the outside of your knee, move your left forearm to the left of your right shin, reach back behind you with the left hand, and bring your right hand around to the left on the floor for balance. It will help bring your shoulders back and your spine straight.

Does the pressure from your right thigh on your abdomen prevent you from twisting any further? Do you find it difficult to twist due to the thickness of your left thigh? As you breathe in, twist your body slightly: then, as you breathe out, straighten up to inspect. As you twist, bring your right hand over your back and to the left to gently pull your right shoulder down and back. To thrust your left chest (not your shoulder) forward and to the right, pull your left shoulder blade back. Is it true that buttock skin makes you wobbly? Does your left arm have trouble passing your right thigh?

If you answered yes to any of the following questions, then mass and size are important considerations. Even if your weight is normal, you may have trouble twisting due of stiffness, a herniated disc, rotator cuff dysfunction, or another injury. You may test whether stiffness or the size of your limbs and abdomen is the limiting factor by doing the same twist while sitting on the floor and while standing with your foot on a chair, like in the first posture above. Get some outside assistance if you feel you lack the ability to judge.

BODY ENERGY, STABILITY, and STRENGTH

Kakasana (The Crow)

Because of the wide range of muscles it engages, this position is a great way to gauge your body's adaptability to meet your changing demands.

Readers in their third or fourth months of pregnancy, or those with osteoporosis, Dupuytren's contractures, or excessive frailty, should refrain from striking this position.

It's not enough to merely test your individual balance, agility, and strength; we need to see how they work together to give you fluid movement and effortless poise. This has nothing to do with your heart health or whether or not you'd make a good Navy SEAL; rather, it concerns whether or not your muscle mass is proportional to your body fat percentage.

Because of the rounded nature of this position, it is not recommended for persons with spinal conditions like as osteopenia, osteoporosis, a herniated lumbar disc, or severe kyphosis.

CONTOURING FOR THE PERFECT STANCE

The Pose

1: Make a soft spot in the centre of a yoga mat with a pillow, a stack of blankets, or any other cushiony object.

2: Step back about a foot from it.

3: Squat.

4: Put your hands about shoulder-width apart. Put your thumbs and index fingers together.

5. Raise your knees as high as you can onto your arms.

6: Squeeze your triceps as you press your thighs inward.
7: Rise up onto the balls of your feet, kicking your heels forward, and shift your body weight forward.
8: Try holding your head up a little bit, but not so much that the back of your neck is being compressed.
9: As you shift your weight forward onto your fingers, lift one foot at a time off the ground. 9. When both feet are off the ground, repeat steps 7-8.
10: This is an excellent place to be. Ten seconds minimum with both feet in the air.

11: The Crow pose, or Kakasana, may be advanced to the Crane pose, or Bakasana, by simply straightening the elbows.
Alternatively, if the Crow appears too difficult to enter, I might suggest a less complicated method. The "liftoff" onto the palms and bent elbows is facilitated by placing a block behind you and stooping down while squeezing your thighs on your triceps.
When trying to strike this stance, what obstacles do you encounter? Weakness in the arms and shoulders in relation to body weight is a common symptom. Having a stomach too big or thighs too heavy to fit onto the upper arms is another possible explanation. The presence of excessive amounts of soft, non-muscular flesh on either the upper or lower extremities makes it difficult to lay one on top of the other without causing instability. Last but not least,

the overall strength-to-weight ratio may overwhelm any semblance of equilibrium.

Here is a risk-free overall evaluation of how well your strength, weight, and balance are in sync, which is especially important if you suffer from osteopenia, osteoporosis, or a ruptured lumbar disc. Those with medical restrictions from trying the Crow pose can instead try the one below.

In this case, the Bridge

It has many positive effects and is a very energising position. It's included in many anti-depressant programmes and is a component of the yoga sequence demonstrated to strengthen bone.

People with spinal stenosis, anterolisthesis, or facet syndrome shouldn't try it. Other conditions that should be avoided include: severe kyphosis, extensive arthritis, late pregnancy, and gastroesophageal reflux disease. If you fit any of these descriptions and are unable to perform the arm balance described above, you may want to take a look at your past activities with an eye toward your overall fitness and consider whether or not you are becoming winded when simply getting dressed to go out or whether or not getting out of a chair is becoming a challenge.

CONTOURING FOR THE PERFECT STANCE

The Pose

1: Lay on your back with a folded blanket beneath your shoulders but not your head. Please keep your arms at your sides.

2: Get on all fours with your knees bent and your feet flat on the floor.
3: .Raise your midsection off the floor, focusing on the area between your belly button and your pubic bone. The kidneys can be supported by placing your hands, palms together, under them. Keep your arms by your sides, and keep your elbows in.
4: Put pressure on your feet with your quadriceps and gluteal muscles as if you were trying to push your feet away from you, but don't do so. Try to get as much of your chest forward over your neck as you can by using the momentum your legs provide to produce forward power and raise your torso and pelvis.
5: Keep your arms and hands where they were; this time, support your upper arch by placing your hands under your lower back, elbows at right angles, and fingers pointing toward each other. Hold the position for at least 30 seconds. Just one minute will do.
6: If you can't accomplish this, if you can't get your belly button to rise, it's a good sign that you need to grow stronger and/or reduce weight. Try this simpler version for a more nuanced evaluation:

VARIATION

Put a strap over your elbows and hold them at shoulder width. Above the elbows, you'll wrap the strap over your arms. Raise your hips and put your hands behind your lower back to do this.

Strength in relation to body weight may be an issue if you can do this but not the strapless version that came before it, although this is less of a concern than being unable to do either.

I've sneakily snuck in three helpful tools for you to use whether or not you need to lose weight:

1: It can boost your motivation by giving you more personal reasons to believe that losing weight is important. You may now see that losing weight might have a major impact on your life, which should increase your drive.

2: Increasing one's belief in one's own power to realise one's goals and actualize one's physical potential. If you've done even a little bit of the yoga here, you've already improved your physical condition. I really hope that you feel more certain about your skills now.

3: After giving yoga a try, you could change your mind and realise it's not as bad as you thought.

Chapter: 4

Real People Get Thinner

It has been argued that yoga's potential to aid weight loss is overstated since it causes your metabolism to slow. I find it ridiculous to assume that yoga has no effect on managing weight. It's true that eating less reduces metabolic energy production and, therefore, calorie expenditure. There are many people and research that attest to yoga's success in long-term weight reduction.

When compared to regular exercise, this has a multiplicity of physiological effects. Our research shows that yoga helps people lose weight, especially when combined with rigorous mindfulness training.

From a biochemical standpoint, yoga has the potential to lessen the production of key hormones like interleukins while increasing the production of others like adiponectin, so facilitating weight reduction and decreasing inflammatory reactions.

I present to you Bryan Wayne, a guy who has been around the block a few times but isn't completely on his own. I've been seeing him since he first came in around seven years ago complaining of back discomfort. He reported that any movement caused pain on both sides of the groove. Bryan spent his days hauling heavy objects like park benches and sewage manhole covers as part of his job with the New York City Parks Department. A "fully filled" description seemed appropriate for him now that he was forty. If you inserted your finger in his stomach, it would come back to bite you. He was obviously arthritic due to his lack of frequent physical activity. His 260-pound frame was disproportionate to his **5'9" height.**

Despite this, he had a sharp mind, was open to new information, and took criticism well. Because of his stiff joints, he listened to me when I told him that the way he utilises his back (which is also tight) is a sure prescription for pain and damage. He said that he had to work harder and had less freedom of movement because of the added burden.

He was unable to reach the large, bushy trees we were planting last week because of his growing belly, he informed me. I couldn't go beneath them because my knees wouldn't bend low enough. There was no

way for me to pick them up and load them into the trolley. I had to haul them across a lengthy expanse of grass. My back aches because of it now. At the moment, the pain is fairly severe.
Jan, a coworker and experienced yogi, kindly took Bryan under her wing and taught him the ropes. The first yoga he attempted was a comical parody that did little to improve his flexibility or range of motion. In order to show him the potential benefits of physical exercise, we needed to get him moving. Jan's enthusiasm for her student's growth was infectious, and after a few weeks, he was no longer blindly obeying her orders. He wanted to recover and experience life with the same uncomplicated joy as Jan enjoyed. The thought struck him, and he went home to try it out.
Twenty pounds and 50% of his back ache gone after just three months. It wasn't long before he joined Weight Watchers. He lost 75 pounds by changing his eating habits and seeing Jan once a week for nearly a whole year. After years of suffering, he was suddenly pain-free and able to practise yoga with some degree of success.
Once again, six months later, I ran into him at a yoga event. He was in excellent form and beaming with happiness. Then he went to see Jan, and he's now thinking about whether or not to add yoga instruction to his busy schedule.

Bryan's success in losing weight because to yoga should not be discounted since he also went to

Weight Watchers, in my opinion. Actually, the opposite is true. There was a Weight Watchers meeting in the area, and all he needed was the inspiration to start going. Shortly thereafter, he was able to let go of his subconscious inclinations and take things seriously, come to grips with the thought that he could, in fact, drop the weight and that doing so would not be such a dreadful thing.

Even though this individual paid close attention to his physical well-being, he did not consider his spiritual well-being. He saw an increase in confidence and acceptance of his physical self after beginning yoga. Even while the physical practise of yoga probably didn't burn as many calories as he needed to reduce weight, it helped him overcome the feelings of shame and disgust with his body, which block many overweight persons from reducing weight.

The physical condition of the participants was also a major factor. Mind-body techniques have been shown to aid in weight reduction, according to research. It's also possible to choose Stacey Morris. With the help of yoga, she dropped 180 pounds and has been able to maintain her new weight for the last decade. Her father and her were "eating friends" as children since they had the same large (okay, overweight) family. The inconsistent eating habits she adopted as a young child just "made her hungry" each time. The continual ups and downs rattled her self-assurance to its core. There was a time when she weighed in at about **300** pounds.

A correction from her: "You are so cruel, oh my god. To have a college flame start saying things like that about me crushed my heart. "What you're doing needs some tweaking. I despised myself more than everyone else. Many women who aren't interested in guys deliberately acquire weight.

She was a journalist for five years while she hid away within her own body.

The 44-year-old lady had created a reputation for herself as a freelance writer who specialised in cuisine, travel, and the arts.

The job was rewarding, but I became stressed out and developed poor eating habits as a result of working in such a hostile atmosphere. The fact that I was confined to a desk for the better part of the day did not help. My intention in writing this was to encourage positive body image. Funny, since I've really written pieces from a similar perspective.

I must confess that I had become too reliant on food. When I was in my twenties, I managed to shed a hundred pounds, only to put them all back on later. Neither of those things helped me feel better about myself. The childhood bullying they endured severely impacted their growth and development. I finally lost my cool and shouted, "Enough!" While being overweight has its challenges, it in no way defines me as a horrible person. To paraphrase my mental monologue: "I can only control what's happening inside; the outside is out of my control."

After then, three more things happened. Beach Boys member Brian Wilson's daughter Carnie has recently been shown on television discussing her battles with obesity. After reading about wrestler Diamond Dallas Page's success with an Ashtanga yoga regimen for weight loss, I decided to give it a go. I weighed a whopping 345 pounds at my heaviest.

Even though I have practised Kundalini yoga for years, I had never heard of this method until now. The spiritual is woven into the fabric of my narrative. Yoga has helped me in so many ways and I highly recommend it. Because of the poor quality of the processed food I was putting into my body, I noticed that I needed much more rest than normal. As my yoga practise progressed, I saw an increase in my vitality, self-awareness, and confidence. A study found that those who regularly practised yoga had a lower rate of biological ageing. Overall, I'm happier and healthier than I was in my twenties.

After getting out of a bad relationship, I retreated to my own company and devoted myself more fully to my yoga practise. I joined a bunch of online dating sites to increase my chances of finding a suitable companion. How fortunate I am to have discovered and been engaged to the woman I've always imagined spending the rest of my life with.

Both gluten and dairy products from cows have lost their appeal to me. I was able to shed pounds without making any other lifestyle adjustments because to yoga. Regular yoga practise helped me shed **20 pounds** in only one month. After that, I stopped always feeling hungry and irritated, and I lost around ten pounds every month. My outlook on my health has been steadily improving. The more weight I lost, the more everything made sense, and now I'm a yoga instructor and author who gives lectures and writes books all over the nation.

Jesse Ruggiere, by age 30, was suffering from arthritis and injured knees in addition to a cardiac condition that required ablation surgery. Thyroid cancer, perhaps caused by Castleman disease, necessitated surgical removal of his thyroid gland. What he ate and drank most of was fast food, Pepsi, and Jack Daniel's. He was 5 feet and 8 inches tall and 236 kg. Jesse's treating physician strongly suggested that he start exercising regularly.

Seeing a YouTube video of DDP (Diamond Dallas Page) Yoga inspired him to realise that if those men could do it, so could he. Over the last six years, Jesse has managed to gain an astonishing 184 pounds. He doesn't drink beer, but he does have six-pack abs. As a spiritual person, I was wondering whether he found any religious significance in his yoga practise. He remarked that the term "spiritual" might have a variety of meanings depending on the listener. I just work out, is how I would put it. In contrast, he claims that yoga has given him a "completely new life." Jesse has made yoga and charity activities like the military-themed Tough Mudder a regular part of his life. For an outing, he brings foster children to their first baseball game. I can think of no other activity that can compare to them on a spiritual level. Really, he seems upbeat about everything. You have the opportunity to improve your health every single day. It's not Bryan, Stacey, Jesse, or anybody else who's been kind enough to share their experiences here. I respect their determination to keep learning and developing in all areas of their being. They are a role model for everyone who struggles with their weight. Knowing that one is not alone is comforting for people who identify with this group. The following are some new findings concerning obesity that may surprise the courageous people who have taken up yoga for its physical and spiritual benefits.

The prevalence of obesity is staggering.

Whether you think it's a major problem or not, if you're having trouble maintaining a healthy weight, you're not alone.

The results of the United States's **2009–2010** National Health and Nutrition Examination Survey revealed:

A staggering **66%** of adults in the United States are either overweight or obese.

Around **7** out of **10** grownups in the United States are overweight or obese.

Almost **20%** of the population is morbidly obese.

More than a third of children and teenagers (**6-19** years old) are overweight or obese.

Half of all kids and teens in this age bracket are fat, according to estimates.

There isn't a reliable way to predict how many yogis are overweight, obese, or severely fat. Maybe you've done yoga before, but I have to ask: Have you ever gone to a class where the bulk of the people were overweight? Sincerity requires me to say that I just don't see that occurring. While there are some men and women who are "large" who still practise yoga, this is by no means the norm. The vast majority fall squarely inside the normative distribution.

Based on data collected between 2009 and 2010, the vast majority of American adults were either overweight or obese (**74%** of men and **64%** of women). One-third of adults of both sexes were obese, with more men being clinically obese than females. Very few men (**4%**) and women (**8%**) were morbidly obese.

The number of overweight and obese Americans has skyrocketed from around a third in the 1960s to roughly two-thirds now.

This is a wonderful idea right here. Yoga is practised by more than **37 million** individuals every day throughout the globe. If yoga is effective in helping individuals shed pounds, as I think it is, it might have a profound and far-reaching impact on the national obesity epidemic.

Chapter: 5

How Yoga Works Deep Inside Your Body

The most compelling reasons for engaging in yoga practise have been discussed. Yogis in the US increased from **20.4%** to **36.8%** of the population between **2012** and **2016**. More than **100** million

Americans practise yoga on a regular basis in their homes. More people practise yoga in the United States than belong to the largest Christian churches. Yes, yoga is now commonly practised by the general public. Not everyone will try it, and that's okay. **Yoga Journal** and the **Yoga Alliance commissioned Ipsos** Public Affairs to investigate the barriers to entry for yoga practise. These top five reasons are presented along with some rebuttals that might sway sceptics.

1: "I'm not sure whether I should do it." However, there is one certain technique to learn the truth.

2: "I have no idea where to begin." The remedy may be found in the book's advice and inspiration. Hold on, there's more reading to be done!

3: "I don't exercise." While holding yoga positions requires quite a bit of physical activity, it is not usually seen as such. Still, you might probably benefit from getting up and stretching right now.

4: This yoga class is not the appropriate setting for me. There are many yoga studios and instructors in the world; everyone should be able to find a practise and instructor that speaks to them. Most of the suggestions in the book may be implemented without ever leaving your house.

5: It's impossible for me to perform yoga since I lack the flexibility required. There are two parts to this question, and each has an answer that there are so many yogis of all shapes and sizes doing yoga now that it's quite improbable that your body is unique. You may have a "non-yoga body," yet yoga practise will nonetheless adapt and change it because of the way it harmonises, coordinates, and integrates you and your body.

When compared to other popular weight loss programmes, yoga's "**side effects**" include **improved posture, balance, range of motion** (ROM), **strength, coordination, anxiety reduction**, and **many more**. Yoga is also easy to learn and practise without breaking the bank or needing any credentials. There is no sophisticated configuration or memorising on your part required. So, I'm wondering how exactly regular yoga practise may aid you in making the change from being a little heavier than you'd want to being a bit lighter.

Your brain and stomach are constantly in communication with one another.

Whether you're wondering if yoga might help you lose weight, keep in mind that, among its many other jobs, your brain also aids in digestion. This provides some insight into the strange eating patterns, lifestyle choices, and physical make-ups that define humans.

Contrast this with the graphic of the human stomach on the adjacent page, which depicts an internal organ and reveals the location of receptors in relation to the brain. The image depicts the acronym "**CNS**," which stands for "central nervous system.

The connection I'm referring about exists not only between the belly and the mind. The first part of the duodenum, the stomach, and the upper oesophagus are all considered to be a part of this system (the first portion of the small intestine beyond the exit of the stomach). The release of gastrin, pepsinogen, and histamine, among other digestive enzymes, occurs in response to a stretch of the abdominal muscles. Muscles in the digestive system are also fortified as a result of this. As the strain increases, however, the body begins to release cholecystokinin and **adiponectin**. Surprisingly, this has the additional effect of slowing down digestion while speeding up the body's fat metabolism. Ghrelin, widely known as the "**hunger hormone**," levels fall considerably. Receptor expansion in the digestive tract, the oesophagus, and the stomach sends signals to the brain's reward and hunger circuits, suppressing their activity. In practically little time at all, you will feel less hungry after doing these stretches. Almost instantly, our hunger subsides. It's possible that some simple yoga postures that focus on the abdominals will aid you in regulating your appetite.

Absorption and digestion are two components of a dynamic system.

To one's surprise, it was found that stretching the stomach from top to bottom had a far greater impact on one's hunger levels than did stretching it from side to side. It may be possible to do this by eating a really big meal or by inflating a balloon within the stomach.

This is achieved by a series of circular breathing and yoga postures that stretch the abdominal area.

Histology, which follows anatomy closely, focuses on the cellular level of analysis, which is found in tissues. Tissues are the super-cellular components of living organisms that exist below the organic level. This describes groups of cells that produce their own special kind of extracellular matrix. Here, we get a detailed look at how a longer oesophagus, stomach, and duodenum affect a person's physiology and their ability to consume food.

Both the hepatoduodenal ligament and the fascia that encircles the head of the pancreas serve to connect the duodenum to the rest of the body. More detail may be seen in the picture beginning on page 35. The usual duodenal arch is somewhat reduced when the two places become apart due of the arch in the back. That is to say, such an elongation falls neatly within the "normal range of motion" for these organs.

The data shown above on the digestive system are the product of extensive research. To spark your curiosity in knowing more about the positive correlation between stretch and slimness, allow me to quickly summarise a few of them. According to studies conducted on animals, increasing one's stomach size is the most effective way to control one's food consumption. Researchers have "removed" this genetic feedback loop that regulates food consumption in fruit flies. These genetic engineering efforts result in enormous fruit flies.

YOUR SENSES AND EMOTIONS HAVE PHYSICAL EFFECTS

Yoga also has this other incredible and related benefit. A heightened awareness of one's environment and oneself develops over time, often without one's knowledge or consent. You are noticeably more aware and awake than normal. This newly discovered sensitivity may be interpreted in two ways: The word "**interoception**" refers to the consciousness that originates inside the body, such as the feeling of movement in one's limbs, nose, or stomach. Exteroception refers to the use of your senses to gather information about the external world, such as vision, hearing, smell, and taste. Yoga's emphasis on improving interoception may explain the unexpected ways in which it might help you lose weight and control your eating habits. Exercising not only has health advantages, but it may also help you control your food cravings.

Research has shown that yoga may boost interoception by increasing one's awareness of internal bodily states and feelings. Here, the yoga helps stretch out receptors that suppress appetite and makes you more receptive to the positive effects of your newly reduced need to eat. Because it focuses on the body from the inside out, yoga may be an effective method of reducing fat.

Is there a mental equivalent to a calorie burn counter at restaurants?

Stress is highly correlated with eating far beyond the typical supper time, and yoga has been shown to reduce stress levels. Late-night snacking has been hypothesised to have a major effect on body mass index by certain studies. Even if it's true that calories are calories, there are other factors to think about.

Midnight is when the appetite-suppressing effect of stretch receptors in the duodenum, stomach, and lower oesophagus is at its weakest, at just **75%** of its daytime intensity. It's not a good idea to go down for a snack at **3** in the morning since you won't be that hungry. You can discover that you're constantly hungry if you're not getting enough sleep and are worried about getting through the next day. **7** The fat-burning hormones leptin and adiponectin are reduced in anxious people, while the fat-making hormone ghrelin is increased. It's never a bad idea to practise yoga to relax.

In addition, studies have shown that the brain is among the body's top energy users. Feeding your body with food that is good for your brain is just one more manner in which the two are interconnected. It amazes me that just around **20%** of our total caloric intake goes to our brains. To better gauge their progress toward enlightenment, some Tibetan yogis accompany their pupils to the snowy mountains to meditate in quiet. In order to understand how yogis can remain perfectly still while still burning calories, we must first determine whether or not they have the power to intentionally stop their hearts.

From the strenuous asanas popularised by **B.K.S. Iyengar** and **K. Pattabhi Jois** to the quiet calm of sitting and standing trances, yoga comprises a wide variety of practises. The cardiovascular and metabolic rates may both increase with some types of yoga (the rate at which food is transformed into energy and exhaled as carbon dioxide and water).

This must be true if you want to successfully shed pounds. Exercise of some kind is a vital part of every yoga practise. Yoga (and other forms of exercise) have been shown in recent years to cause cellular changes that help with weight management. Modern research has proved beyond a reasonable doubt two of these alterations, one occurring inside the cell and another in its nucleus.

More mitochondria are preferred if weight loss is a goal.

The protein known as **peroxisome proliferator-activated receptor gamma coactivator-1alpha** (PGC-1alpha) has a boring name, but it's a formidable intracellular warrior that helps prevent diseases including arthritis, inflammation, Alzheimer's, heart disease, and numerous types of cancer. It has been discovered to increase the proliferation of fat-burning mitochondria in the human body. 9. Since mitochondria are the most potent ally, if not the sole ally, of all of us who desire to lose weight, it makes sense to teach you a little bit about them. PGC-1alpha, a protein, is the most potent stimulator of mitochondrial replication. Mitochondria originated from a symbiotic connection between a bacterium and an animal cell. We may safely assume that the current age of Earth predates the start of this process by at least a billion years. Mitochondria are often thought to have originated in an undigested bacteria that was taken in by an animal cell. Thus, it could exist solely inside the mammalian cells. Following an initial adjustment period, the bacterial

DNA began fueling the animal cell, providing it an edge over its competitors. Only these cells that had been strengthened by bacteria and their offspring survived. In animals, the larger cells have found a method to work with the smaller bacterial cells inside them, with the bacteria providing more energy and the larger cells safeguarding the internal power stations from outside influence.

With the evolution of mitochondria, cells were able to specialise, leading to the development of the liver, the retina, and other marvels of coordinated activity characteristic of sophisticated animals and humans. DNA can be found in both the nucleus and the mitochondria, but neither can work alone. Proteins encoded by DNA in the nucleus are crucial for mitochondrial function. But the DNA in mitochondria is what produces the structures that provide almost all of the energy the body needs. Greater numbers of mitochondria are seen in cells with higher energy demands. An estimated **2,000** reside in each liver cell. Estimates suggest that mitochondria make up around **40%** of heart muscle. Ten percent to twelve percent of a person's bulk is made up of mitochondria.

Mitochondria are the cell's power plants.

Each and every one of our molecules relies on electricity to power its machinery. Our nerves and muscles operate similarly to electrical lines and motors, however our muscles act more like ratcheting than spinning electric motors. Only inside mitochondria can electrons be transmitted.

Furthermore, the greater our number of mitochondria, the greater our strength. More energy is generated from glucose when PGC-1alpha is produced at a faster pace. By doing this, you will be able to lose weight and feel more energised.

In PGC-1alpha-induced mitochondrial proliferation, there is some indication that mitochondria, like the bacteria they evolved from, may spontaneously cluster together and divide. To continue its vital function once DNA or other components degrade or get damaged, a mitochondrion will find a method to merge with a healthy mitochondrion. Internal cell systems trigger mitochondrial division when a cell need more energy. The natural world, as is so often the case, provides strategies for preserving balance. Furthermore, forces formed inside of each cell regulate mitochondrial growth and production. Rather, PGC-1alpha is the essential component in raising their numbers.

What does this indicate for dieters who want to reduce their body mass index?

When mitochondrial number rises, metabolic rate follows suit. The liver's ability to generate glucose, metabolise it, and release lipid-breaking enzymes increases in direct proportion to the amount of mitochondria it contains. When there are more mitochondria present in cartilage cells, the joint is better protected against the degenerative effects of arthritis. There will be positive effects on your tendons, immune system, thyroid, memory cells, and the reward centres of your brain. You'll experience a boost in productivity across the board. You can lose weight by burning more calories than you consume each day, provided you do it in a method that doesn't negatively impact your health or fitness. Mitochondrial enrichment is the only way to make such a dramatic improvement. While doing yoga, your metabolism slows down, but regular practise increases energy expenditure. You may as well say that getting a college degree doesn't help you make more money because you don't get paid to go to school, since that's the logic behind the assertion that yoga doesn't help you lose weight because it slows your metabolism. Instead, you may put the same effort into yoga and find that it helps you live a richer, more satisfying life.

Most physicians will say something like, "Your metabolism slows down as you grow older" to explain away the weight gain that is common in middle age. Less selective sensory perception leads to less sensitive hunger centres, which is only one of the numerous causes leading to this alteration in so many people's bodies. However, with the help of more mitochondria, all these abilities may be restored to, and even surpassed by, those of younger individuals. Yoga may temporarily slow your metabolism, but its fat-burning effects are long-lasting because of the hormone PGC-1alpha it triggers. In the long run, mitochondrial proliferation is the consequence. The efficiency with which your cells transform food into energy, your metabolic rate, and your body fat may all be enhanced by adding more mitochondria to your cells.

TELOMERES

While this is true, there are other ways in which yoga aids in weight reduction. Sadly, the opposite is usually the case. In all multicellular organisms, the priceless DNA instructions that teach each cell what to be and do are stored in strands of repeating DNA. The repeating telomeres at the ends of the chromosomes protect the unique sets of instructions that decide whether an egg will hatch a pigeon or a trout. Each cell's nucleus contains chromosomes that contain critical instruction lists that are held in place by telomeric DNA strands, much as a kite's tail holds the construction aloft when the wind picks up. Sailing in gentler seas calls for a longer tail.

In the midst of the calm molecular whirlpool that is cellular life, telomeres act as a rock to protect your DNA. There is an increased risk of cancer, decreased generation of thyroid hormone, worse digestion, and other DNA dysfunctions with ageing because telomeres shorten with each cell cycle. Telomere shortening is an important factor in the ageing process. 11

According to current knowledge, telomere length is the sole genetic trait that may be affected by an individual's manner of life. The length of your telomeres may be affected by factors like as your stress levels and coping techniques, diet, amount of physical activity, and happiness, all of which may be passed on to your offspring. The length of the telomeres in your inherited DNA may be affected by your social network, the trustworthiness of your friends and coworkers, and even your location.

While there is currently no study that focuses on hatha yoga and telomeres, it has been proven that yoga, along with tai chi and qigong, may help decrease inflammation and oxidative stress, both of which are known to shorten telomeres. Also, telomerase, the enzyme that mysteriously lengthens your chromosomes' protective caps called telomeres, is boosted by meditation. Whether you're into the mindfulness taught by **Jon Kabat-Zinn** or **Deepak Chopra's mantra-filled meditation retreats** or the **more conventional meditation** used by the majority of Americans, this holds true. All of these methods have the potential to modify gene expression in a manner that reduces cellular stress and inflammation, according to the data currently available. These mechanisms mitigate the rate of telomere shortening and, in certain instances, prolong telomeres on the cell's nucleus DNA.

A further benefit of telomeres is that they may be lengthened without extreme efforts like starvation for a week or a regimen of thousands of push-ups every day. On the other hand, longer telomeres have been associated with a positive outlook on life, an absence of stress, and a feeling of purpose.

"**Healthspan**" is defined in the book The Telomere Effect by Nobel laureate Elizabeth Blackburn and her colleague Elissa Epel as the length of years over which a person's cells cycle normally, led by longer strands of telomeres, and so demonstrate a majority of healthy tissues.

They cite studies that indicate how the number of years a person is sick or dying rises in the latter half of their lives (their "**diseasespan**"). The writers of this piece make a compelling case for the role of telomere shortening in the onset of chronic illness and eventual mortality. Immunity, skin and intestinal lining regeneration, memory, and virility are just few of the many indicators of young that are connected with telomere length. Your telomeres' length is inversely proportional to how long you live. In addition, there seems to be a correlation between telomere length and lifespan.

Blackburn received the Nobel Prize in Chemistry for his work in discovering telomerase, an enzyme that encourages the extension of telomeres. Telomeres, which serve as a protective cap at the end of each chromosome, may be lengthened by the enzyme telomerase. To what do you attribute this potential increase, and why? Reducing stress, improving one's outlook on life, and practising yoga on a daily basis are all terrific places to start. Those who become negative, hostile, or insecure in the face of adversity have much shorter telomeres than those who react well to stress. Activating telomerase and lengthening telomeres is more common in optimistic persons and those with high stress tolerance.

Central to a yogic way of life is the practise of meditation. Since it is common knowledge that regular meditation reduces stress, and since reduced stress benefits in weight reduction, there is no need to elaborate. Biochemical evidence supports this claim, which brings us to number fifteen. From the metabolic mechanism in each of our billions of cells to the ends of the chromosomes that predict our lifespan down to the most basic, feet-on-the-scale level, we have shown this to be true.

Now is a great moment to look at how yoga may help you lose weight specifically. One neurophysiological mechanism by which yoga reduces appetite is the stretching of the gastrointestinal system, which activates receptors that carry inhibitory signals to the brain's reward and hunger centres. Apples may replace sausages as your preferred snack meal if your preferences shift slightly.

Brown fat cells increase in number as a consequence of regular yoga practise, outnumbering white fat cells (which are more resistant to being burnt off) The metabolic rate of a cell is proportional to the amount of mitochondria it has.

Moreover, I think it's crucial to mention that yoga is a superb method for relieving tension and unwinding. Hormones like norepinephrine are released in reaction to common sources of stress, such as a tardy teacher or gridlocked traffic. These hormones promote the demise of certain cells by increasing their oxidation rate. In most cases, this is a bad plan. Yoga, however, seems to activate telomerase and even make it by providing the optimal kind of exercise that enhances the body's performance.

Chapter: 6

Motivation, Medical Risks, Drugs, and Diets

According to a recent research, adding connections to additional objectives can increase a person's drive to complete the primary objective. Knowing that one's hard-earned money will go toward pleasures such as paying off debt, sending children to college, or updating living room furnishings may inspire a person to work more. 1. People like Nathan Pritikin and Dean Ornish, MD, introduced the public to nutritional innovations in the 1970s. Since then, people have come to understand that there are many more advantages to maintaining a healthy lifestyle than just looking nice. Increased body fat negatively impacts cardiovascular health. However, an increasing number of people aren't driven to improve their health by the promise of future generations, the want to look good, the desire to keep diabetes and heart disease at bay, or the desire to delay the onset of arthritis. Incredibly low levels of motivation like this are hard to fathom. If someone's health is in jeopardy because of their weight, I believe it's crucial to find strategies to push them to reduce weight. To what extent, if any, does reducing body fat improve one's quality of life?

Because of the numerous good impacts yoga has on one's body, mind, and spirit, I'm writing this in the hopes of inspiring others to give it a try. According to a local, "even the devoted no longer believe in God" in New York City. Since I am not an expert in this field, I will refrain from offering my opinion. Nonetheless, my own experience and that of my students have convinced me that yoga's nontheistic but palpable spirituality raises one's awareness, concentrates one's thoughts, softens one's attitudes, and ultimately permeates one's very being. The very fact that you are able to read this shows not only that you are alive, but also that you possess the potential for spiritual growth apart from the guidance of the world's major religions. In my opinion, doing yoga regularly may add several years to your life expectancy.

The mental and spiritual benefits of yoga go beyond what can be achieved via diet and exercise alone. Practicing yoga helps hone one's sense of identity until it more closely corresponds with the Buddhist teaching that all things are interrelated and the profound proclamation of B.K.S. Iyengar that "your body is your temple." Yoga's innate holiness, in addition to its well-documented physiological advantages, may help us see the sanctity of every area of our lives.

As a whole, the goal becomes more apparent: you want to inspire people to take action by making them feel enthused about doing so. Practicing yoga regularly may improve not only your physical health, but also your interpersonal connections and your capacity to enjoy nature. This allows you to concentrate on your own aspirations and to confront your own concerns squarely. Yoga is beneficial since it encourages introspection, which is something that can only help one's health. Practicing yoga has been demonstrated to improve cognitive function, cardiovascular health, and spiritual well-being, and it also seems to have some kind of esoteric resonance with the human body. Let's put all our persuasive energies on getting you to and keeping you at a healthy weight and level of mental acuity. It is my duty as a doctor to stress the positive effects of moderation on one's health.

Culture and historical period have a significant impact on what is considered a healthy weight. Whether you're in sixteenth-century Holland or modern-day Jamaica, the idea that larger is better is universal. Most of us adopt a "**to each his own**" attitude to problems of taste. However, in the twenty-first century, we cannot just take a dispassionate, subjective look at our physical selves and remain mentally inflexible. There is no way to conceptualise the brain and the rest of the body as two distinct entities. The distance between the mirror and the scale is bigger than the smallest variation in attractiveness that can be seen by the human eye. Our ever-changing surroundings include not just our social interactions but also our self-awareness and the direction in which we see ourselves developing. Expertise may also be gained through the scientific community's researchers.

For What Reasons Do Doctors Urge Patients to Lose Weight?

Most of us don't need to be reminded that having a high BMI is dangerous, any more than we need a warning label with a skull and crossbones to know that smoking cigarettes is dangerous. Increases in obesity prevalence represent a true public health crisis. No other words can express it adequately. Let me try anyhow.

Diabetes

Nearly all of America's nearly **26** million diabetics are overweight. Statistical estimates suggest that at least **7** million individuals have diabetes but don't realise it. As much as **95%** of all diabetes cases are attributable to type **2** diabetes. More than **90%** of patients with type **2** diabetes are either overweight or obese, making obesity a significant risk factor for getting the condition. Even a modest weight decrease of **5** percent may have health benefits due to the correlation between obesity and type 2 diabetes.

High blood pressure, stroke, retinal disease, coronary artery disease, neuropathy, many pregnancy difficulties, oral health concerns, and even certain kinds of **leukaemia** have all been linked to diabetes. Diabetes is a leading cause of amputations, blindness, and kidney failure.

Several cancers, including leukaemia and melanoma, may be more difficult to cure if patients are overweight, suggests a new research. The death rate from diabetes is twice as high as the national average for persons of similar ages. Diseases related to diabetes are the eighth largest cause of death in the United States. The risk of death from any cause increases almost linearly in European countries if blood sugar levels go above **100 milligrammes** per deciliter.

Obesity is linked to an increased chance of developing prediabetes. After the age of 45, the frequency of prediabetes skyrockets, affecting half of those over 65.

Arthritis

The foot, ankle, knee, and hip sizes of a person seldom vary significantly between the wearing of a belt size 26 and 36. Every extra pound you carry puts more of a strain on your bones and joints. Arthritis affects one in five Americans, but it affects three in five overweight people.

People who were overweight or obese had a reduced chance of success with conservative treatment and even surgery for arthritis. Some of the biochemicals linked to obesity have also been shown to cause inflammation, and this may be why. One possible source of the harm that being overweight brings, particularly to the joints, is that "excess adipose tissue creates humoral chemicals, altering articular cartilage metabolism," as one British research puts it. People who are overweight or obese are more likely to suffer from chronic inflammation, which may contribute to the development of or worsen existing arthritic symptoms. When there are more humoral components in the blood and interstitial tissues, the body produces less of the powerful anti-inflammatory protein PGC-1alpha. Our results show that low levels of PGC-1alpha also impact mitochondrial activity, which in turn disrupts the normal functioning of your cells, especially those crucial for the maintenance of bone and cartilage.

PGC-1alpha protects against a wide variety of diseases while being as common as water. Another research verified the link between gout and arthritis, this time emphasising the involvement of humoral mechanisms beyond mere physical pressure on the joint, and a British investigation validated the link between fat and knee osteoarthritis. For now, however, let's speak on arthritis rather than the advantages of yoga.

Since arthritis, especially when compounded by the additional stress of being overweight, may make it difficult to move about, it is crucial to consider postsurgical rehabilitation soon after the operation. Despite a few outliers, research has consistently linked BMI to increased postoperative pain and impairment in individuals who have had total knee replacements. Patients who are overweight have a more difficult and protracted recovery after knee surgery. However, there are occassions when a little extra muscle is useful. Some plastic-surgery treatments have a mortality risk that is twelve times greater in morbidly obese persons, despite the fact that cardiac surgery is more difficult on the very thin and that fatality rates drop with rising body mass index.

Illnesses affecting the heart

Having a body mass index (BMI) more than **30** indicates obesity. There are people in this category who are at least **5 feet 8 inches** tall and **200 pounds** in weight, and others who are shorter (but still over **175 pounds**) at **5 feet 4 inches** tall. Because of the disproportionate share these cases have in the country's healthcare costs, researchers have paid close attention to them. What we may learn from them may be generalizable to a larger population of overweight individuals who do not yet meet the criteria for the severe category.

Heart disease, sleep apnea, pulmonary hypertension, stroke, coronary heart disease, congestive heart failure, and arrhythmias are all more common among obese and overweight adults, as is their chance of death overall. Compared to slimmer individuals, those who are overweight have a **sixfold** increased risk of having hypertension. Although habitual joggers who are overweight are likely healthier than their non-jogging peers, they nonetheless have a higher risk of a heart attack or stroke than their thinner running friends. It was previously reported by a doctor practising in a rural region that some of their patients would eat their own flesh before taking their own lives.

MOOD

But there's something else about being overweight that could be even more important than the rest: a lack of optimism. Nobody knows for sure if the medical difficulties, the many biochemical or mechanical consequences of being overweight, or the modest but widespread cultural stigma connected to severe obesity account for the disproportionately high incidence of depression recorded among the overweight. This is contingent on a wide range of other variables. In the age-old chicken-or-egg dispute, there are two schools of thought: Is morbid obesity a symptom of depression, or a possible cause of it? **Possible explanation**: the social disgrace associated with being overweight in today's society.

No matter the root of one's pessimism, the end effect is a failure to take charge of one's own life. The English word "despair" accurately describes how you feel right now. Nobody ever wakes up, leaves their house, and finds themselves homeless that same day. One of the strongest correlations between pessimistic perspective and weight gain is the opposite.

Because of my extensive background in this area and my dedication to staying abreast of cutting-edge research, I am confident in saying that you can successfully lose weight if you put in the time and effort required. The weight of despair and sadness may be lifted when one takes action and sees positive results. Weight loss is the polar opposite of a slippery slope. There is still a link between being overweight and being unhappy, even after controlling for things like chronic pain and physical illnesses.

Other Options

There is a way out of the loop of binge eating, guilt, and depression, and you can win the game. Please know that you have my complete backing if you decide to give it a go.

DRUGS

These days, it's easy to find a weight-loss pill to help you in your quest. That in itself should be a red flag that the current course of therapy is less than ideal. However, despite the potential for great chemical diversity, they may be roughly classified into two categories: Amphetamines are one kind of drug that may reduce hunger while simultaneously increasing energy expenditure. It's possible that if the other group were to only intervene in that one mechanism, it would be enough to prevent further fat storage. Eliminating a football player's access to PEDs is analogous to the first kind. His ability to build muscle and exert physical force is going away. The second group is using a strategy that has the same impact as taking off a single conveyor belt from an assembly line, namely a decrease in output.

The primary advantage of systemic medicine is that it causes fewer serious adverse effects. The widespread nature of their impact raises concerns that it might negatively affect people's health. One benefit of drugs with a narrower therapeutic window is that they have fewer adverse effects and, thus, improve patients' quality of life.

Those with system-wide influence: In 2016, the **FDA authorised Qsymia,** a timed-release combination of the popular weight-loss medicine phentermine and the anti-convulsant and migraine headache treatment topiramate (an appetite suppressant and metabolism accelerator). Paraesthesias, dizziness, insomnia, and a changed sense of taste are just some of the neurological side effects that have been linked to phentermine, a substance chemically related to amphetamine. Other common complaints include dry mouth and constipation. Yet these are merely the most widely recognised drawbacks. There are numerous adverse effects, including harm to the developing foetus, diarrhoea, psychomotor delay, memory loss, and yellowing of the eyes.

Consequences of being overweight have been studied extensively. Trading these benefits for something else might be a step backwards. Drugs that are equal to or superior than those currently on the market tend to get approved by the FDA. The approval of a treatment that fits this profile allows us to speculate about the potential dangers and benefits of similar medications that came before it.

Another drug that contains phentermine is called Suprenza. Without the risk of adverse reactions, the tale remains the same while using topiramate. Possible adverse responses include dizziness, weakness, swelling in the ankles and feet, high blood pressure, weariness, headache, foul taste in the mouth, changes in sex desire, and impotence.

Saxenda is unique in its field. Glucagon-like peptide-1 (GLP-1) is a protein with wide-ranging physiological effects, and its active form is called GLP-1. In a nutshell, it reduces hunger by keeping blood sugar from dropping too low and reducing the rate at which food is discharged from the stomach, both of which limit the rate at which the intestine can break down the meal. These signs and symptoms may all be brought on by a lack of appetite.

Since yoga does the same thing in a noticeably different way: by activating the gastrointestinal (GI) stretch receptors, yoga tricks the body into thinking it's just eaten a full meal. Possible side effects of Saxenda are listed below. Thyroid tumours, both benign and malignant, were seen in laboratory mice and rats. Thyroid tumours, suicidal thoughts and actions, hypoglycemia, and the classic vomiting, nausea, and diarrhoea have all been linked to it in people. Alternatively stated, yoga is completely risk-free. However, it has been used successfully to treat a variety of these ailments.

The antidepressant bupropion is combined with the opioid antagonist subutex to create Contrave (naltrexone). It has a nicotinic impact and is chemically related to amphetamine, which has been used on occasion to help smokers quit. Possible negative reactions include hypoglycemia, naltrexone-induced liver damage, antidepressant-induced angle-closure glaucoma, and suicidal ideation or behaviour (particularly concerning given the correlation between obesity and depression).

To provide just one example, consider the drug Xenical, which has its desired effect by inhibiting a specific metabolic pathway. It competes with digestive enzymes for access to dietary fats, which is how it achieves its peculiar effect. By doing so, fatty molecules are blocked from entering the circulation via the gut wall. One advantage of medicine is its narrow therapeutic window. The effects of Xenical are limited to the stomach's digestive cells and processes. The enzymes in question must be blocked significantly for Xenical to have any impact. It's hardly surprising that it causes gastrointestinal symptoms including **diarrhoea, bloating**, and **gas**.

The time has come to end this pharmacological discussion. You should weigh the benefits of each against those of yoga to decide which is best for you. If you want to lose weight, gain weight, or simply ignore the issue and go to the movies, the illusive bluebird of happiness will decide. According to research including **163,066 Britons**, being overweight is dangerous, and depression in men is also strongly associated with poor health. A decrease in happiness and health was seen for both sexes when body mass index climbed.

One thing sticks out when thinking about the studies done on these medications. Some medications may have somewhat different directions for use, but they all stress the need of sticking to a calorie-restricted diet and doing regular exercise. Because of this, it is likely that the doctor will also suggest that the patient make some lifestyle changes, such as modifying their diet and increasing their level of physical activity.

Going on a guilt trip about the hazards of obesity to a reader who is on the point of giving up hope might be motivated by ulterior motives. The correct amount of weight-related criticism might motivate you to make changes. This entails receiving just enough constructive criticism to spur you into action, without absorbing so much that you become paralysed by guilt and despair. In this part, we'll make our second pitch for why you should follow through on what you already know to be the best course of action. Also, it provides evidence that this aim is feasible via yoga.

However, two courageous clinical researchers have a lot to credit for the success of any alternative weight reduction method. They specifically affected the treatment of cardiovascular disease and the obesity that contributes to it. There are a few people whose names stick out in my mind: **Dr. Dean Ornish** and **Nathan Pritikin.**

It is possible that Nathan Pritikin, then a young engineer just starting out in the field, was the first to conceptualise input-output correlations as a way of conceptualising heart disease. Patients with coronary artery disease who followed his low-fat diet and exercise plan saw improvements. Dean Ornish, who advocated for stress-reduction techniques like yoga and meditation, is a possible analogue. Their work has led to a heightened awareness of apparently mundane parts of everyday life that have been shown to have far-reaching health consequences.

These two individuals may be seen as the originators of the present preoccupation with **gluten**, **GMOs**, **supplements**, **the paleo** diet, the Mito diet, the Whole30 diet, and even (to an extent) yoga. The

concepts presented here, including yoga, complement the benefits gained by eating healthfully and engaging in almost any kind of physical exercise. As our knowledge of the human genome increases, individualised eating programmes may one day be possible. In the meanwhile, know that they are but concepts.
Many individuals who lose weight by cutting calories regain it within two to three years, despite their boasts of accomplishment.
In many cases, the causes of the yo-yo effect remain a mystery. Kevin Hall's research at the NIH shows that individuals who lose weight are able to maintain their weight loss for a time, but eventually hit a plateau and regain the weight they lost. It's not uncommon for people trying to lose weight to resort to drastic measures like cutting off carbohydrates or sweets. Given how difficult it is to keep to such drastic dietary changes, many of us resort to gradually reintroducing the items we were so eager to cut out in the first place, convincing ourselves that we won't gain weight if we eat just a little amount. After being without it for a while, a few pieces of bread may not seem like much. A single one will ensure that they don't. Losing weight is facilitated by including them back into your diet on a regular basis. In addition, one popular strategy is to monitor one's calorie consumption. Most packaged food calorie counts are inaccurate or understated. Consequently, it's very feasible that even the most meticulous calorie trackers are missing some food.

Proteins and carbohydrates are digested differently, and processed meals are either eliminated or retained differently. There is no difference in the total quantity of calories among these foods, but they all have unique storage and cooking requirements. Regardless of whether or not we monitor our caloric intake, we must never lose sight of the role that our genes play in dictating our final body composition. The risk of becoming overweight has been proven to have a heritable component by researchers. An individual's obesity risk score has the potential to be used as a BMI predictor.

Clearly, further study is required, but at the same time, we are only scratching the surface of understanding how the bacteria in our gut may affect our health, and in particular, our ability to gain or lose weight. Individual differences in the duration and intensity of positive and negative emotions, as well as the ability to regulate one's own eating, exercise, and sleep patterns, all have a part in one's ability to successfully lose or gain weight.

Fortunately, we are shifting our attention from the total number of calories to the quality of the meals we consume. Both regular exercise and a diet high in whole, unprocessed meals and a spectrum of colourful vegetables help minimise weight fluctuations.

Despite our best efforts, diet medications have been widely accessible for quite some time. Multiple of them have sophisticated biological systems.

Contrary to common belief, some may actually boost **leptin** levels, which are associated with fat loss. The use of amphetamines, for instance, has been linked to changes in appetite. It's possible that the way you eat will be changed by the medicines you take because of the way they affect your physical functioning. Diet pills may be effective in the short term for weight loss, but they usually have serious adverse effects that make them unsafe for long-term usage. **Garcinia cambogia**, a fruit native to Southeast Asia, has gained popularity as a dietary supplement in recent years. Those who struggle with "emotional eating" may benefit from trying this since it reduces hunger and boosts serotonin levels (also known as the "happy hormone"). However, there are also potential drawbacks to using such supplements. There has to be more study done to establish that these supplements do not aid in weight reduction. A condition called liver necrosis may be brought on by using garcinia cambogia.

Some weight reduction plans put an emphasis on limiting calories rather than physical exercise, despite the fact that the former has been shown to be more effective at promoting long-term weight loss. Consumption-reducing yoga complements the other three methods. The two could work better together.

Expanding one's focus beyond the act of eating

1: By paying greater attention to your food while eating and savouring its aroma, flavour, and texture, you may find that you feel fuller more quickly. Focusing on each step of the eating process, from choosing to preparing to finishing your food, might help you feel full more quickly and regularly. Meals cooked at home are just as good as those served in restaurants.

2: There are two fundamental mental shifts required to significantly reduce caloric intake. It's important to keep in mind that there are **7.8 billion** big species on Earth, all of which consume food and produce waste on a regular basis, and that human actions have an influence on this fragile ecology. Our donation of **$7,801,000** is a big sum. If we can find a happy medium between consumption, nutrition, and recycling, maybe the situation will improve.

3: you should adjust your diet to incorporate more healthful foods. Following the Whole **30** plan necessitates a **30-day** period during which participants abstain from eating any foods containing sugar, alcohol, wheat, dairy, legumes, peanut butter, carrageenan, MSG, sulfites, or baked or processed goods. To assist you reach your weight loss goals, various diets use various tactics, including meal planning, calorie limitations, lists of disallowed items, and reward programmes.

Some diets are healthy because they activate mitochondria, like the Atkins, paleo, Mito, and keto diets; while others, like Hyperfit, include pre-cooked meals that are intended to help you lose one to two pounds per week (e.g., SlimFast). Whereas, meal

replacement plans like Medifast and Nutrisystem limit how often you may have alternative meals delivered to your house.
People with diabetes, who may benefit most from a particular diet, have many alternatives to select from. I wholeheartedly recommend The Diabetes Diet by Dr. Richard Bernstein. A professional dietitian or nutritionist may assist you in creating a personalised food plan. The need of consuming vitamin, mineral, and electrolyte-rich meals is emphasised by several of them. If you're looking for a food plan tailored to your blood type, Eat Right for Your Type is the only book available.
Perhaps what differentiates Weight Watchers from other comparable programmes is its emphasis on points rather than calorie counting. Weight Watchers' success may be attributed to its many tasty and nutritious food options, as well as its focus on motivation, use of social pressure, and group support sessions. producing no unfavourable outcomes or adding any unnecessary dangers. Thanks to this method, a friend of mine who had struggled with her weight since she was a kid is now at her goal weight.
In conclusion, diets deserve praise for their ability to effectively demonstrate the dieter's control over his or her body weight. Many individuals have found, to their joy, that they can successfully control their weight by altering their diet. It's not simple to keep the weight off, even if you plan your meals wisely and exercise often. No matter how motivated you are,

dieting alone won't be enough to keep you on track with your weight reduction objectives. And here is where it most diverges from yoga.

SURGERY

To lose weight, you may also use a gadget that squeezes your stomach. After the surgeon has removed tissue from the pouch, either traditionally (by stitching) or via the use of balloons, the pouch's size is decreased (a more recent method). It's too soon to tell how effective balloon methods are, but if surgery is necessary, surgeons need to be mindful of preserving the satiety-inducing receptors and **enterocrine glands**.

All of these strategies affect both the kinds and amounts of food consumed, as well as how well those foods are absorbed. It has nothing to do with food, and especially not the pressures and rewards associated with eating. One of the most obvious benefits of yoga is this. I was able to meet Marcie Hammond via my involvement with the Beach-body group. Marcie works as a wardrobe assistant in the company's video-filming division and attributes most of her weight reduction to yoga.

I sometimes go back to when I first began practising yoga and wonder how much more I weighed. In the last two years, I have gone on many diets and have dropped a total of sixty-two pounds. Half of the funds should be returned after two years. The change in hormone levels following menopause is associated with a decrease in mood. I put on 50 pounds because of menopause. Losing and winning have always occurred in alternating cycles for me. To this day, I still don't know what triggered my sporadic weight fluctuations. I felt like my body was about to collapse at any second, yet my intellect was as sharp as ever. The mental aspect of weight gain is crucial. Nothing of this sort can be physically grasped. The human race has an innate need to eat when stressed or upset. That's how I've felt on the inside for as long as I can remember.

My go-to method for venturing into unknown territory has always been yoga. I needed to go in because, without it, I was feeling worn out, disappointed, and hopeless. In my mind, only the really slender and limber could pull it off. After three weeks of yoga at Beach Body, I realised that I always have the skills necessary to succeed. Stress and anxiety are supposedly reduced and serenity is attained via yoga. It would be difficult to find something better for one's mental health. I was at the end of my rope, so I decided to give this a go. At my lowest point, I thought there was no hope for me to ever get better.

I felt like a phoney and a failure because of everything I had lost and then gained in those two years. In order to achieve my goals, I decided to practise yoga. tremendously scary. Although I found the original methods to be too difficult, I found that the adapted versions were quite helpful. I was only able to execute shaky, half-hearted stretches as a consequence. Three weeks of class time with the instructor. We met for class three times a week and used DVDs to complete homework at other times. Compared to other diet plans, this one was completely novel. I was getting to the meat of the issue by taking stock of my own psychological and emotional state. helping me accomplish my goals and preventing harm to my health. I want to improve my diet even more so I can reach my goals.

The same regulation applied to our food supply. Maintaining a healthy diet, practising yoga, and sorting out my thoughts. I was able to reduce the dosage of my antidepressant. I was ready to crash the moment I got home. I was able to concentrate much better. My chest congestion has eased. Slowly, the realisation of a strategy for calming down came to me. About five months ago, I began a regular practise of yoga.

In recent years, my yoga practise has become so integral to my daily life that I can't imagine functioning without it. Everything I've tried from this brand has helped me immensely. Yoga helps me get ready for the day, so I do it first thing in the morning and last thing at night. Now my body and brain are under control. Also, I want very much to keep my current weight. The relief from menopausal symptoms, insomnia, and stress-related binge eating is incredible. It was as if the introduction of yoga had been meticulously planned.

In the past, I'll admit, I was a junk food addict. Healthy food isn't something I naturally enjoy, but I'm trying to improve my relationship with it because I know it's vital to my well-being. Why that wouldn't

be useful is beyond me. I've learned that eating just once a week sets me up for despair and binge eating. Your actions are harmful to your health. Therefore, once a week, I give myself a reward. I don't beat myself up, no.
Meditation became common after yoga became popular. That's useful, thanks. If I feel myself becoming anxious, I take a minute to centre myself via deep breathing and meditation. I'm not only not eating, but also not medicating. Wish I'd known about this sooner. As I took in the bunch of young, waiflike pretzels, I knew I'd never fit in. Alternatively, I've never been more flexible than I am now. Many of us have issues controlling our emotional eating during menopause. When I should have been focusing on my mental health, I had been worrying about my body.

Chapter: 7

Doing the Yoga

Through yoga, you will gain a new appreciation for the world around you. You'll see the same benefit in your body. This will silently, and maybe even without your notice, bring about huge changes in your life. The earliest, subtle changes in how you feel and see the environment will pave the way for more substantial adaptations in the future. As a physician who has treated many patients over the years and as a man who has practised yoga regularly for forty years, I say this without reservation. Yoga is spiritual but not religious. The similarities between its moral guidelines and the Ten Commandments are unsettling. Yoga, like many religions, may help you have a more enlightened and liberated perspective on the world. In contrast, yoga does not need any kind of initiation fee or clergy to practise: a yogi is someone who does yoga. Finally, that's it. That's how simple it is. Even if yogic beliefs have spiritual roots and are intended to benefit humanity, they cannot be accepted credibly without regular yoga practice.Yoga is connected to your day-to-day mental and physical activities, and it promotes restful sleep. However, a spiritual purpose serves as its primary motivation.

This might be the most convincing evidence that yoga has against becoming overweight. Your sense of your own sanctity will grow. It separates the enjoyable from the outstanding, giving you strong motivation to seek out the former and avoid the latter. This is a universal characteristic of all religious endeavours. However, physical actions are an integral part of yoga. It drains your devotion to everything but what is beneficial for you and the world, leaving you with the motivation and drive to go for that. It's imperative that you practise yoga.

The knowledge of human anatomy and physiology that we gained in **Chapter 5** is a good place to begin. As we have said, there are several yoga poses that target the abdominal area and its contents. There is a direct connection between the stretch receptors in the duodenum, the stomach, and the esophageal sphincter and the brain regions responsible for hunger. The tenth cranial nerve, or vagus nerve, includes sensory fibres that pick up signals and send them to the nucleus solitarius, which in turn connects to the hypothalamus, the nucleus accumbens, and the arcuate nucleus, all of which have a significant effect on the desire to eat. Reduced hunger may be achieved by the activation of the body's stretch receptors, which can be achieved through the stretching of yoga postures or by filling one's stomach to capacity. Some yoga poses specifically target and strengthen these areas.

When learning a new technique, it's best to begin with the simplest positions and work your way up to the more complex versions only when you feel comfortable doing so. You'll be doing exercises that may help you burn calories while learning about the refined and elegant inner workings of your body. This peculiar but natural bond will illuminate your life with spiritual clarity, allowing you to appreciate the sacredness of your own body and mind.

General rules while practicing yoga

1: Exercise in a well-lit, flat, clean, and secure area.

2: Calm down to broaden your perspective and maintain more control.

If you've never done yoga before, it's best to get some guidance from a professional so you can get started on the right foot.

3: Learn as much as you can about the relevant anatomy.

4: Imagine the stretch receptors sending signals to suppress hunger.Visualizing what is happening within and outside your body while practising the postures may be an essential tool, similar to how familiarity with the streets of a city may be used to get around more easily.

5: Give each pose a good go only once, and then move on to the next. There's no need to beat yourself up about it since there will be another chance to do better.

Remember the person or people who have meant the most to you in your life.Treat yourself with the same kindness you would provide for a friend.

When possible, take a five-to fifteen-minute break after completing the whole sequence of postures. Take a minute or two of quiet, focused relaxation per hour.

6: Perform the exercises when your stomach is empty or nearly so.

Don't practise yoga for at least three hours after eating; wait four or five if you're over 55 or have stomach acid.

To make sure you can safely do the pose, first review the warnings. Except as otherwise stated, the relative contraindications are minimal. A skilled and resourceful teacher may help you find an alternative job that offers similar benefits to the one you can't do because of your health. Typically, a scaled-down variant, a variant that makes use of aids, or a work-around will suffice for the same purpose. Even if you learn the poses at a different time of day or in a different class, the best time to practise them for optimal results is fifteen to thirty minutes before a meal.

A yoga mat, a belt, and a block are the typical accoutrements. Chairs made out of card tables or chairs with a similar design might be useful as well.
Don't push yourself so hard that you're in serious agony. Although yoga has healing properties, it also has the potential to do harm. Tense muscles are normal after exercise (although do it with caution) (although be careful). The goal of yoga practise should be to gain mastery, not to let go. Stop the pose and go to a yoga teacher or doctor if you feel any pain. If you're just starting out, start with the easiest moves and work your way up to the more advanced ones when you're ready.

ASANA

Although all the postures are beneficial for weight loss, some may be more comfortable for you than others. To get the most out of your practise time, you should experiment with different postures until you find the ones that work best for you. The potential side effects are the biggest red flags. They're shown before the instructions for each stance to make it clear when it's not a good idea to strike that pose. It's best to get started with the roles that don't have any major drawbacks preventing you from giving them all your attention right away. Those benefits will increase as your inhibitions melt away.
Honor your needs while making full use of your skills. The backbends are designed for those with an exceptional range of motion. If your lunchtime weight gain is the main issue, you may have to do the poses at your desk at work, where you have little

choice but to stand up. If you're having trouble keeping your balance, try the seated postures first. Ensure proper form before executing the postures with conviction. Regularly doing the postures for three to four weeks before eating, namely fifteen to thirty minutes beforehand, has been shown to be effective. Perform a pre-and post-time interval weigh-in. Feeling more confident in your abilities and the outcome of your efforts as the number on the scale decreases is natural and expected. I think you'll find this helpful since yoga has the potential to be a reliable and trustworthy companion for the rest of your life if you give it the chance.

There are several reported benefits to many common yoga postures. As an example, forward bends are great for relieving hamstring tightness and spinal stenosis. When there is a major benefit that is generally applicable, it is highlighted in the body of the posture's description. The additional benefits may help you choose which poses to practise on a daily basis when you have mastered a variety of postures.

1: STANDING

The best you can do is stand there at times.

When you have hip arthritis, have a hip replacement (posterior approach), have a herniated disc, piriformis syndrome, or can only do yoga in the bathroom.

2: When you are unable to take a seat because of anything other than your own choosing then try Tadasana, that thing up There.

Who among yoga practitioners hasn't been instructed to strike a pose meant to evoke the living tranquilly of an immovable mountain? This posture requires the practitioner to be strong and focused while maintaining a state of equilibrium. Who hasn't stood, their skin tingling with the unfamiliar sense of attentive calm, aware of the powerful, even surge of calm inside their own bodies? When one remains still, the sense of self-awareness is heightened.

Implications and usage: This is a great example of how even small amounts of self-control can pay off in spectacular ways. Without having to actively do anything, breathing naturally slows down, ushering in a wave of mental and bodily calm. In addition to highlighting the benefits of good posture, self-reliance, and individuality, this stance highlights the joys and responsibilities that come with having a body.

Contradictions:

Foot, ankle, knee, or hip flexion contractures; extreme leg-length discrepancy; severe imbalance; advanced congestive heart failure; and chronic venous insufficiency are all contraindications.

THE STANCE

1: Stand with the fronts of your feet shoulder-width apart.

2: Raise your toes, spread them apart, and then put them back down to increase the surface area you're standing on.

3: Feel the ground beneath you with the thin stems of your toes.These stems are located between your foot and the fleshy tips of your toes.
4: Split your body weight in half on each foot, for a total of 12. The proper placement is six on the heel, two on the big toe, and one on each of the other toes and metatarsal heads.
5: Align your ankles, hips, shoulders, and ears by shifting your pelvis, shoulders, and neck.
6: Keep your gaze steady and your mind open to new information.
7: Let your mouth's soft and hard palates loosen up.
8: Lengthen out, namely at the back of the neck and the shins.
9: Allow your fingers and thumbs to be thick enough at the tips to expand your hands and reduce stress on your cuticles.
10: Take a minute to focus on your breathing, and be sure to do it softly, evenly, and in both directions.
The benefits and mechanism of action are as follows: better posture causes the oesophagus and anterior stomach to enlarge. As such, it acts as a mild appetite suppressant. The accomplishment of this deceptively simple pose—a test of balance, flexibility, and coordination—can inspire a sense of pride and independence. Although it may take some time to perfect, practitioners of this art are proud to adopt the lotus posture as a sign of and a show of their independence and grace after they have mastered it. Furthermore, it presents a safe challenge and gradually enhances balance. In addition, the posture

strengthens bones by stimulating osteocytes and applying pressure in both the vertical and horizontal planes to the hips and spine. Increased awareness, focus, and symmetry are all benefits.

Ankle instability, severe rotator cuff syndrome, plantar fasciitis, peroneal palsy, subacromial impingement, and poor balance are all conditions that should be avoided.

Tips that may be of assistance: Looking intently at a point level with your eyes, expand the front and sides of your rib cage as you raise your arms overhead, stretching them as far as possible, and distribute your weight evenly across your standing foot (**50 percent on the heel**, **25 percent on the big toe**, and the remaining **25 percent on each of the lesser toes** and **metatarsal pads**).

The Classic Pose (Variation Flow)

1: Spread your toes and stand with your feet hip-width apart. Put all of your weight on your left foot by pressing down on the ball and heel. Firm up your whole left thigh by gently contracting your quadriceps and hamstrings. You may gradually stretch your hip by bringing your lower pelvis forward. Your lumbar curve should be reduced using these methods.

2: Place the shins directly above the hips. Raise your right foot so that it rests on the top of your left thigh, with your toes pointing toward your left ankle. If your lower leg doesn't reach that high, try resting it on your calf instead. Try not to rest it squarely on your knee.

3: Keep your pelvis pointing forward while bending your right knee and bringing your right leg out to the side (ideally at a ninety-degree angle to your left foot) (ideally at ninety degrees to the left foot).
4: Drop the right leg lower, stretching the quadriceps, if your right hip is now higher than your left. In most cases, that will help restore balance to the hips.
5: Move the lower pelvis forward to re-open the hips. Target an object fifteen to twenty feet in front of you and bring it back into focus.
6: Inhale as you raise both arms over your head in a symmetrical manner, bringing the palms together in front of your face and the biceps as far back behind your ears as you can get them without craning your neck. Relax and fill your lungs to capacity before proceeding.
7: Bring your shoulder blades close together behind you; reach upward from your left ankle to your finger-and thumbtips. Lift your foot off the mat so that just the skin is touching the floor.
8: Repeatedly inhale and exhale slowly in a symmetrical pattern for 8 minutes.
9: Exhale and drop your arms when you reach number 9.
10: Perform 10 slow repetitions of lifting your arms and inhaling deeply. Gently lower your body until both feet are flat on the floor. Legs should be switched and the process repeated.

VARIATIONS

1: Standing with your back against a wall, brace the chair's side against the wall so it faces you. Toes pointing away from you, rest your right foot on the chair's seat. Then proceed as described above. This is a sensible and secure way to begin testing your balance on one foot, and it is also a strategy for beginning to expand the gastrointestinal system. The slow process begins when you lift your right foot off the chair and gradually shift your weight to your left foot. This is a lot more challenging than the standard position,. but it's much safer.

2: Do the position without a chair against a wall. The right heel should be tucked into the left's shinbone or into the left's lower leg. It's still a secure position to be in at this time.

3: The act of propping up one leg with the other will undoubtedly cause a tightening of the abdominal muscles and the need to readjust one's posture. The answer to suppressed hunger can be found here.

4: Creating a vertical arch in the back stretches the lower oesophagus, the whole stomach, and the duodenum, which all contribute to a decrease in appetite. Herniated disc pain is alleviated as a result of the partial vacuum created at the fronts of the lumbar and thoracic vertebral bodies, which pushes the herniated disc material forward. In doing so, the disc material is pushed back down where it belongs, under the vertebral bodies and away from the nerve roots.

5: Dislocation of the knee joint (especially of the anterior or posterior cruciate ligaments); severe plantar fasciitis; Achilles tendonitis; extreme weakness; central spinal stenosis;

The structure

1: Jump with your feet spaced four and a half feet apart and your arms extended, palms facing upwards. Take a deep breath in and out and calm down.

2: While keeping your arms at your sides, turn your right foot out ninety degrees and your left foot in thirty degrees.Stand with your legs completely straight and your pelvis rotated 90 degrees so that your left hip faces forward and your right hip faces back.

3: Squat down such that your right shin is perpendicular to the floor and your right thigh is parallel to the floor. Put your whole weight on the big toe of your left foot as you pivot your torso to the outside. To counteract this pull and maintain the forward position of the left hip, weight should be borne on the ball of the left foot.

4: Raise your thumbs and index fingers.

5: Relax for a full minute by breathing normally.

Reversing the sequence of steps 1 through 5 will put you back on your feet for step 6. Always put your left foot forward for the next five steps.

For people with weak or shaky legs, there is Virabhadrasana I, or the chair pose.

VARIATIONS

1: With your left leg bent and parallel to the back of a chair, rest the back of your thigh on the seat. Keep your left hand on the chair's back for support, and put your right hand on your crooked leg. Get out of the chair slowly over the course of a week or more as your confidence increases. Use your thighs rather than your arms for this. Extend your arms to the side or even up over your head if you feel stable enough to do so.

2: Support your front leg with a block while in the classic posture. It also lifts the body and rocks it backward, which stretches the digestive system and helps the less flexible spine get into an upright posture. This posture may be simplified by taking a wider stance, in which the legs are not in a straight line, but doing so eliminates the therapeutic effects.

BACKBENDS

By far the most energising postures, and possibly the most effective at suppressing appetite. Though I describe these positions as helpful for herniated discs in my book Healing Yoga, I caution those with spinal stenosis, anterolisthesis, or facet syndrome to stay away from them. Third, these postures are especially helpful for those who are overweight because of the increased occurrence of ruptured discs in this population.

Keeping your body in the right position is crucial. As you repeatedly put your body through these motions, it will eventually become comfortable in them. These first positions, which may be rather challenging, need to be held for ten to twenty seconds. Ideally, you'd want to start with a small amount of time and work your way up to a minute or more.

Salabhasana
The Locust

By blocking impulses to the nucleus solitarius and other reward centres in the brain, stretching the anterior oesophagus, stomach, and duodenum reduces hunger. Efficient in bolstering the whole collection of back extensors.

Herniated discs cause low back discomfort for many people and are especially common in overweight persons. A partial vacuum is created in front of the disc by separating the vertebral bodies above and below it, therefore reducing pressure on the disc and easing the disease. The herniated disc is repositioned between the vertebrae, where it belongs, and the nerve roots that are emerging from the spinal canal are protected. Holding this position for long periods of time may help you build strength in the muscles that maintain your back arched (**quadratus lumborum, multifidus, iliocostalis**, etc.). **Spinal stenosis, spondylolisthesis** (**anterolisthesis**), facet syndrome, and pregnancy beyond the first trimester are among disorders that should be avoided

THE BUILDING

1: Have a horizontal upper torso and hands at your sides. Moving clockwise from the head: the neck, the solar plexus (the region right between the ribs), the hips, the toes, and the cuticles.

2: If you need a little more support, you may use the area between your Adam's apple and the insides of your knees. Stretch your Achilles tendon and the back of your neck.

3: Inhale as you raise your arms parallel to the floor, palms down; repeat (a) and (b) once more, this time with your hands on your hips and your ankles gently squeezed together (b). Put your mind at ease and give your body a good long stretch, focusing on the front.

4: The recommendation to tense one's abdominal muscles may appear paradoxical at first. To a certain degree, you may lessen the arch by drawing them tighter. If your stomach is flat, like a "flat tyre," you may be able to go farther and faster without being as hungry.

CHANGES THAT CAUSE MINIMAL DISTURBANCE

1: Press your palms together at your shoulders and lift your upper body. In this case, you must maintain your torso still and your gaze down. If you lean back too much, you risk hitting your head. Don't ever stare at the other person straight in the eyes; rather, tilt your chin up instead of your forehead.

2: Posture is enhanced by stretching the lower chest, and the oesophagus, stomach, and duodenum are lengthened, stretched, and relaxed by arching the thoracic and lumbar spines. The lower oesophagus, stomach, and duodenum are compressed more forcefully, while the upper oesophagus, along with the surrounding neck are kept still. Reflux esophagitis, cervical disc herniation, significant kyphosis, advanced arthritis, late pregnancy, and lumbar spinal stenosis are among medical conditions that should be avoided.

THAT BUILDING

1: Lay on your back and tuck the folded end of a blanket under your shoulders, avoiding your head. Position your feet flat on the floor, parallel to one another, and kneel down.

2: Tighten your quadriceps and press down on your feet as if you were trying to push off, but don't really do it. Use the power your legs provide to get your body and pelvis off the ground, and then thrust your chest as far forward over your neck as you can.

3: Lean on your forearms for support, elbows at right angles, fingers touching.

4: Take a few calm, deep breaths, filling your lungs all the way from the bottom up, around your diaphragm and kidneys, and then up and forward into your upper ribcage.

5: You'll want to place your whole weight on your feet while also lifting your hips and bringing your chest closer to the vertical.

6: To relax the oesophagus, stomach, and duodenum while stretching, one should release tension in the pelvic diaphragm and anal muscles.

7: Spend a full minute or more there, number seven. Please let me know if you have a minute to talk.

Variations with fewer Totally Unachievable Benchmarks

(Blankets in a similar position)

1: You may achieve the same result by lying on a bolster, a big cushion, or many blankets if you'd rather not raise your body's trunk.
2: Place a brick or two under your sacrum for support, then push up to sit up straight.
3: Place a strap across your chest and over your upper arms, keeping your elbows at your sides. The strap works best when placed on the upper forearm, but may be worn elsewhere if preferred. Place your hands beneath your lower back for more support as you lift your pelvis. Using a circular motion, the stretches will work to strengthen the abdominal muscles.

Ustrasana
Similar to a camel

This method's advantages and processes lay in the fact that it expands the full digestive system as opposed to just a piece of it, and that it does so more effectively than other techniques. The small intestine winds around the abdomen in an irregular fashion for approximately 28 feet, providing enough "slack" and eliminating the risk of ripping, breaking, or fraying. The omentum and the gastroduodenal ligament, which holds the lower stomach and the beginning of the duodenum in place, are the sole structural connective tissue that bind the whole tract together, therefore some tension will be created.
When a person with a herniated disc bends forward from the waist, the disc material is pushed forward and away from the nerve roots due to the partial vacuum formed between the front parts of the

vertebral bodies. The spinal cord is able to adapt to areas of compression by following the global curvature as it gradually leads it upward through the vertebral canal and toward the skull.

Spinal stenosis, anterolisthesis, anterior labral tear (hips), severe arthritis, carotid or vertebral artery disease, late pregnancy, anterior cruciate or meniscal tears, and chondromalacia patellae are among conditions that should not be treated in this manner.

THE FRAMEUP

1: Keep your feet a little more apart than hip-distance and your knees slightly bent as you stand. The toes have distinct angles. We need to take a breather from the fast pace.

2: Don't clear your throat or strain your tummy when you reach back to grasp your heels.

3: To do this, lean forward from the hips and shoulders, and rest your weight on the backs of your hands and heels.

4: The gentle rearward lean of the head is the fourth posture. Your health might benefit greatly from even a moderate degree of hip mobility.

5: You can go forward into a palm-up stance by steering with your toes and stomping with your heels. Instead of using the quadriceps to assist raise the pelvis, the hamstrings might be employed. If your neck is rounded, your mouth will be jutted out as well.

6: Relax and allow your chest rise as you let out a deep breath.

7: If you find that you are unable to take a full breath via your nose, consider taking a few large gulps of air in through your stomach instead. By doing so, you will be able to expand your rib cage and take a fuller breath.
8: Bring your upper back and shoulders down toward your stomach to exhale using your diaphragm.
9: Stay in this posture and take 30-60 slow, deep breaths through your nose.

Effort-reducing adjustments

1: Kneel in front of a chair with your shins parallel and your lower back placed on the front of the chair. The toes have distinct angles. Place your palms down on the chair back with your fingers pointed behind you. Put your hands behind your back and lean back in your chair. Let your guard down and lean back.
2: Rest in the supine position with your legs propped up on a thick pillow. Lift your hips and upper body off the cushion by driving up through your heels.
3: Many people who attempt Ustrasana make the error of tensing their quadriceps, which leads to an excessive extension of the knee and a subsequent collapse of the arch. The groyne crossing on the pelvis is unique to the rectus femoris of the quadriceps. When this muscle is contracted, the angle between the pelvis and the thigh is actually reduced, the opposite of the intended effect. Using your hamstrings and gluteus maximus while resting your quadriceps and abs may help you develop and strengthen your arch.

4: Finalize the posture by sitting back between your heels and walking your hands back, away from your feet. To get into this position, bend your elbows and drop your lower back to the mat (Supta Virasana). To do this, stand tall with your feet hip-width apart and your arms at your sides, palms facing up and elbows locked. To do this, just lie on the floor and extend such that your head gradually drops away from your shoulders. You may need help from a teacher or a friend to bring your torso to the floor if this is a new position for you. Supporting your upper body using cushions or a bolster will allow you to lay comfortably face up on the mat with your arms stretched out.

5: Moves forward with twists and turns.

6: These postures compress the abdominal organs, providing a condition of muscular balance that decreases appetite in response to backbends, which create an increase in abdominal size by constricting the dorsal region. Someone suffering from spinal stenosis may find relief in these yoga poses.

Since bowing is not required under all circumstances, the word "bow" should be used figuratively. When this happens, the whole body stoops forward, head first. When the intestines are stretched beyond their usual range of motion, they prolapse from their dorsal, or back, position. Posterior to the fundus and extending into the pyloric antrum is a dense concentration of nerve fibres that transmit signals.

Those who suffer from IBS, a herniated disc, a torn hamstring, or osteoporosis should avoid this exercise.

Sitting on a pile of folded blankets may help those who have problems bending at the hips.

Janu Sirsasana
(Head-to-knee pose)

The structure

1: To start, choose a flat area in front of you and sit down, spreading your legs apart.

2: Lean forward from the waist and cross your right ankle over your left knee. Your right foot should always be in an absolutely vertical posture.

3: Line up your shoulder blades with the tops of your feet.

4: The agonist-antagonist reaction is triggered when the right quadriceps are contracted, which in turn relaxes the hamstrings and glutes.

THE FRAMEUP

1: Do something as simple as crossing your legs in front of you every morning to start your day off right. It may be helpful to fold a blanket and use it to encourage a forward pelvic tilt when seated, and you may do this if you discover that doing so is comfortable.

2: You should next draw your buttocks and upper thighs back after spreading your fingers. Then, moving the pelvis forward is aided by pressing the hands down into the mat.

3: Inhale deeply, filling your lungs to the brim, and exhale slowly; this will cause your upper back to arch. The quickest method to stand up is to press your hands down on the floor next to you.
4: Lie flat on the mat on the inner (medial) or outside (lateral) of the left thigh with the right knee bent.

5: Extend the sole of your left foot as far as it will go and hoist yourself up onto your left leg. Get your foot out by placing your whole weight on the outside edge of your big toe.
6: Turn to the right as you exhale, then straighten your spine as you inhale.
7: The left shoulder must be rotated outside the right knee during the seventh movement. You should keep your right arm in a straight line.
8: Drag the belly button in and up, and then exhale to twist even farther. Beginning the twist from the bottom left side of your rib cage and rotating those ribs to the right is ideal.
9: Wrap your left arm in front of your bent right leg and across it so that your left hand is pointed in toward your left thigh.
10: Clasp your hands or cross your right arm over your left hip to increase the stretch even further.
11: For a deep inhale, lift your right arm above and rotate your right shoulder back and up. As you let your breath out, rotate to the right, bringing your left chest forward and pushing down with your left foot.
12: Inhale evenly and exhale slowly while holding this position for 12 deep breaths. Turning on the twist

helps the listener focus while also calming them down. There's a chance that giving your stomach a little twist to the right may give it a break. Turning to the left might help alleviate stress by making the stomach feel full.

13: After a little interval, do it once again, this time starting on the other side.

Paschimottanasana
(Extreme forward bend)

1: Put a blanket over your thighs by folding it in half. This will result in a forward tilt of your pelvis. Put your feet up and relax, knees out in front of you.

2: Next, use your hands to pull your buttocks and upper thighs back and apart, which will further advance your pelvis.

3: When you exhale, your chest will expand and your spine will stretch, placing you in a prime position for action. Get your shoulders down and back, and put your hands flat on the floor next to you to achieve this.

4: Put your right foot down on the mat next to your left leg while bending your right knee.

5: In order to accomplish step five, plant your left foot firmly on the ground and extend your leg all the way through your sole. Get your foot out by placing your whole weight on the outside edge of your big toe.

6: While keeping your spine neutral and taking a big breath in, rotate to the right.

7: The seventh movement is to place the top part of your left arm outside of your right knee while stretching the forearm vertically. Put your right hand on the floor for balance and push the outside edge of your knee with your elbow to bring your shoulders and spine into a neutral position.

8: The eighth movement is to raise your right elbow and drop your right shoulder as you go behind someone with your left hand. It's possible to do this by bending forward at the hips and bringing your left chest forward with the aid of your left elbow.

9: While doing so, curve your spine inward and take a deep breath; for extra emphasis, raise your right hand to the tips of your fingers.

10: Let your breath out as you twist even farther.

11: If you have a tendency to round off on one side, take deep, even breaths and focus on evenly expanding your chest on both sides.

12: When the referee calls "change legs," both teams must swap.

Paschimottanasana
(Extreme forward bend)

If you slide your right hand under the back of the chair, you can get to the arm on the left side. Reduce the amount of movement in your knees and hips.

The fourth motion occurs on an inhale, when the chest and shoulders are lifted.

In this position, as you exhale, you should move your upper body forward gently, bending your elbows until you feel a gentle stretch along your spine.

As you exhale, clasp your hands and rotate once again, this time placing your left arm over the back of the right armrest and your right hand over the

back of the left chair. In the sixth place, when you breathe out, sit down, and when you breathe in, stand up.
As a rule of thumb, you shouldn't carry yourself with your shoulders rounded forward.
After a count of two or three, keep your back, chest, and right shoulder completely straight as you let out your breath.
Just turn the table over and give it another attempt after waiting a minute.
Stand in a triangle with your legs up (Ardha Matsyendrasana).

The Fish Lord Launches an Attack

Marichyasana III benefits the digestive system by stretching the duodenum, stomach, and oesophagus, and this benefit may be amplified by bending the straight leg, which elongates the thigh.
By adopting this posture, you may get relief from bone loss.
If you have a herniated disc in your lumbar spine (unless you can rotate to the other side), a rotator cuff injury, severe scoliosis, ankylosing spondylitis, rods or wires in your spine, a vertebral fracture, or a colostomy, you should not do this exercise.

The structure

1: The beginning posture consists of sitting on a blanket folded in half with your legs stretched out in front of you.
2: Put your shoulders back and expand your chest. Because of this, you will be less likely to slump over.

You'll experience a rearward change in bone alignment as a result of this adjustment.

3: The next move is to stride out with your left foot beyond your right hip and bend your left knee so that your shin and knee are looking forward. Keep your shins perpendicular to the ground as you bend your right knee and plant your right foot flat on the floor just outside your left thigh. Holding the right knee with both hands is the proper posture.

4: As you inhale, press down on your pelvic bones and up on your spine towards the very end of the breath. Even if you already know you can't, you should attempt some isometric exercises to see if you can increase the space between your thighs nevertheless. Keep your back in this posture as you prepare for the twist.

5: To do a right twist, hold your breath for a few seconds, then exhale as you bring the left side of your belly button in and the tailbone sinks. Raise your left hand and forearm over your head and bring your left elbow around the outside thigh of your right knee.

6: While inhaling deeply, is to reach down with your right hand behind your back and touch the floor.

7: The seventh is a fantastic opportunity to take a large breath in and stretch your back and chest out. Exhale completely and further twist such that your right hand is behind your left shoulder.

8: Check out the eighth listing over on the right. Sit up straight with your head and spine in a neutral posture.

9: To find a secure posture, check that your pelvis is distributing the weight of your body evenly between your two legs.
10: Maintain a state of calm and steadiness by taking a few deep breaths while you look in the new direction. While the discomfort in your back and ribs will make any significant inward rotation impossible, you may be able to execute a little amount of rotation.
11: Take a deep breath and pivot around to go back to face your right knee.
12: If you want to seem neat and put together, don't cross your legs but rather maintain them together at hip level in front of you.
Simply do Step 12 once again on the other side.

13: When you have done both sides and sat for a few minutes, you will begin to feel the benefits of this position all throughout your body.
14: The thoracic spine can only rotate in an extended position. Don't forget to constantly lead with your hips. Engage your ab muscles to help you twist.
All of the upper digestive system is stretched and twisted, with the highest effect felt at the gastroesophageal junction, where many stretch receptors are located, as most of the twisting action occurs between T12 (the final rib-carrying vertebra) and L1 (the first lumbar segment) (the first lumbar segment). Some people get relief from buttock pain (also known as piriformis syndrome) by assuming

this position. If you want to walk without wobbling, balance your weight evenly between your feet.
It's important to note that not everyone agrees that it's vital to flex the buttocks as far as they'll go and scissor the thighs together. When the hips are in a perpendicular position to one another, the sacrum may do part of the twisting, relieving pressure on the lumbar spine and hips. To get the most out of this move, you should do one large, full-body twist that starts at the back of the heel of your supporting foot and extends all the way up to the nape of your neck. As a result, the twist will be more evenly distributed around the body, leading to greater stability and a "safety valve" that may be used to strengthen a vulnerable area. However, locking the thighs at a ninety-degree angle is important when the sacroiliac joint is displaced or when a posterior hip replacement is being done.
Pregnancy beyond the second trimester, a colostomy, a herniated lumbar disc, a dislocation of the sacroiliac joints, and severe spinal (facet) arthritis are all reasons to avoid this procedure.

The structure

1: Stand with your feet shoulder-width apart; bend your right knee to a right angle (90 degrees) and your left knee to a left angle (30 degrees).
2: Make sure your feet are hip-width apart, and your arms are at your sides with your palms facing down.
3: De-stressing is step number three.
4: Place your left hand on the floor or a block next to your right foot as you exhale (little toe side).

5: Get your shoulders back and down and lengthen your spine.
6: Strive for a straight line from your hips to your shoulders as you do this exercise.
There will be less fat all over your body and your upper body will seem longer.

VARIATION

1: The first thing you should do is position your left foot at a 30 degree angle toward the wall as you face the wall and put your left foot close to the ground. The correct foot placement is four inches out from the wall, perpendicular to it.
2: Hold your arms out in front of you with your palms facing down.
3: The next action is to twist diagonally to the right, bringing the left arm over the head and down to the outside of the right foot.
4: Position your left hand such that your big toe is next to your little finger. If the right hand is unable to reach, the left might be utilised to grab the right foot or ankle.
5: If even that seems too much, you may always hold your hand up on a chair or a block.
6: Turn around till your right side is against the wall, then lean against it and touch your right shoulder blade.
7: If you put the palm of your left hand on the floor, your ankle, or a chair, you can maintain this posture safely.

8: The eighth and final correct move is a scissor motion with the legs. Lengthen and slim down completely.

9: Lengthen your body, starting at the back of the knees and working your way up to the top of your head.

10: For the next 30 seconds, number ten, please remain seated. Remember to breathe steadily and slowly.

11: Repeat the procedure, this time beginning at Step 11 with your back against a wall.

12: This is the Jathara Parivartanasana, to be exact.

13: Flip over into a prone posture.
The key benefit and mechanism of action of this position is the elongating impact of the twisting motion on the digestive system. Coordination between the low back (the lumbar region), sacrum (the pelvic base), and hips (the thigh region) is essential for optimal performance. The risk of getting arthritis may be lowered by avoiding practises that prioritise the care of one joint over another. It strengthens the abdominal muscles all the way from the transverse abdominis to the obliques and lateral obliques. Furthermore, after switching to this posture, the agonising pain of facet syndrome, from which I had been suffering, has abated. The torque

exerted by the position on the lumbar vertebrae is considered to be sufficient to enhance bone mineral density, however there is no research to back this up at the time of writing.

In the latter stages of pregnancy, it is best to prevent disorders like trochanteric bursitis, colostomies, herniated lumbar discs, aortic aneurysms, and sacroiliac joint derangement.

That structure

1: The first thing to do is to lie flat on your back.

2: Keep your feet hip-width apart and your arms at your sides, palms facing outward.

3: Inhale deeply and stretch your hands and feet as wide as possible.

4: try bending forward at the hips and knees to a 90-degree angle while exhaling.

5: Finally, make sure your legs are as straight as possible, like two planks of wood.

6: Asana (Tadasana) is the second part of the Mountain Series, from which the Lotus Pose (Supta Padangusthasana) follows (Jathara Parivartanasana).

7: Lower your left buttocks to the floor and squat.

8: As a seventh step, bend your knees to the right and put your feet close to your hands.

9: Raise your left arm and look at your shoulder. The right hand and arm will do the trick to bring your complete back flat on the floor.

10: Stop moving for a full minute (one minute on each side).

Note: Asana called "Halfway there" or "Jathara Parivartanasana" in yoga.

Keep your body in the "Plow" position (Jathara Parivartanasana). This is the Jathara Parivartanasana, to be exact. Jathara Parivartanasana, or "The Side-to-Side Pose," entails a turn to one side during the transition (a less strenuous variant of the pose).

Modifications that won't rock the boat

1: The first thing to do is to lie flat on your back.

2: Keep your feet hip-width apart and your arms at your sides, palms facing outward.

3: Inhale deeply and reach as far as you can with your extended heel and the back of your hand.

4: Make a 90-degree angle with your hips and knees as you exhale.

5: Jut out your left buttocks.

6: Gently lower your right leg to the floor while you raise your knees to your forearms. If you are wearing a heel block and your heels are not touching the ground when you walk, you should stop doing so.

7: Knees should be as straight as possible. Maintain a little bend in your knees to reduce the risk of damage; as your skills develop, you may straighten them. It's similar to the rheostat on a light switch in that it allows for fine adjustment of the illumination.

8: In a moment, you'll notice that your left shoulder is raised somewhat. If you push down on the palm of your right hand, your whole body will crumple to the floor.

9: Try to keep that position for at least 30 seconds.

10: Continue until you have exhausted both possibilities.

These yoga poses are the only ones shown to help you lose weight safely and effectively, so make them your first stop. Concerns that are warranted about them, and about yoga in general, should now be our priority.

The correct way to bend forward at the hips while keeping the back straight is as follows:

Bend at the hips, not the neck, if you want to go down on one knee. You should take your gaze away from your knee and put it on your intended foot placement.

Create the cross sign by putting the palm of your right hand on the inside of your right foot's arch and the palm of your left hand on the inside of your left wrist, then releasing and repeating the gesture six times.

Remain in that position for 30-60 seconds as you concentrate on slow, steady breathing. The next step is to swap the legs around.

VARIATION

To reach the feet, a belt may be wrapped over the straight leg's foot. Start by grabbing the belt with both hands, then securing it by sliding your fingers forward and locking your elbows. With a rowing motion of the shoulders, the head may be brought forward toward the foot instead of down and out toward the knee.

Advantages:

There are three advantages to working here. It does this by putting pressure to the sciatic nerve, the hamstrings, the adductors, and the gluteal muscles, activating the numerous sensory nerves implanted inside the muscles, and therefore sending powerful signals to the areas of the brain that reduce anxiety and hunger. Because of the bending forward motion, the spinal cord is pushed down within the spinal canal, closer to the lower body. Benefits of spinal cord activation treatment can include a general sense of calmness. This may be a helpful posture for those with spinal stenosis since it allows the spine to splay out a little.

Discourages:

Discouraged participants include those who have had a herniated disc, ostomies, or a total hip replacement (posterior approach).

Folding from the hips might be difficult for some people, so doing this while sitting on a folded blanket may help.

The structure:

In order to sit comfortably, you should:

1: spread your legs out in front of you and bring your inner ankles together.

2: Pull your shoulders back and deep breath.

3: To finish the third step, release your breath and bow forward from the hips. A belt over the feet, buckle over the arches, and a hand on each ball of the feet are two options for this.

4: Maintain a relaxed, natural stance with your arms at your sides and feet together, toes tucked in toward your knees (toes not pointed).
5: Rather of hunching over, consider the fifth posture instead: placing your knees beneath your face (if you can reach it).
6: Heavy enough elbows will draw you down; at this point, you may relax the muscles in your thighs. When in pain, it might assist to take it easy and consciously inhale several deep breaths.
7: If you place your palm on your stomach while bending forward, the weight of your hand will assist pull your organs back and down while the foot of your bent leg rests under your rib cage. This will cause the whole duodenum and stomach to enlarge. Poor posture, such as **hyperlordosis** and **kyphosis**, is a common trait among the obese. Obese people often experience stiffness in the hamstrings and lower back muscle spasms. In fact, this posture will help you feel lighter in the legs and less tension in the lower back. The bent leg stretches the quadriceps and hamstrings gently yet efficiently. The strong quadratus lumborum muscles are stretched and relaxed by the forward pull of the arms and abdominal muscles, as well as the pressure of the lotus foot on the abdomen. The triceps, which are responsible for extending the elbow, automatically relax when the biceps are used to bend the elbow. One of two paired muscles will tighten in response to a contraction in the other. In any kind of this role, it

is advantageous to possess the capacity to both inhibit and be inhibited.

You should put off surgery if you are pregnant, have severe arthritis in your knees or hips, have recently broken your ankles, or have a history of osteoporosis.

If you're trying to stand on one leg, you should put the foot of your "**lotus**" leg as far up on the thigh of your "straight" leg as you feel stable doing so. The Lotus Position. A tiny bend in the knee helps you to go farther than you would if you attempted to keep the leg completely straight, since you are sacrificing part of the reciprocal inhibition between the hamstrings and the quadriceps. On the other hand, if you bend forward, you may stretch the quadratus lumborum muscle in your lower back while also sating your hunger. Inhibitory reflexes are activated at maximum extension, and after 30-60 seconds, the hamstrings relax.

"gives a powerful pull on the navel and abdominal organs," as yoga master B.K.S. Iyengar puts it.

The structure

1: To begin, assume a seated position with your left leg extended and pointed upward. Shoulders and upper body should rotate such that the back is horizontal.

2: Place the heel of your right foot on the middle of your right lower abdomen and bend your right knee. If you take a deep breath in, hold it for a second, and then exhale, you may feel better.

3: As a third bend forward at the hips rather than the waist as you walk.

4: Option four is to hold your left foot in both hands or reach across your body and grab your left wrist with your right. Instead of pulling your chest in, push it out. Relax your shoulders and straighten your elbows. Rest on your bent elbows and let gravity carry you forward.

5: By leaning forward and then backward, one may assume the "half lotus" pose (Ardha Baddha Padma Janusirsasana).

Modifications that won't rock the boat

Get the loop at the sole of your shoe ready for your belt. Stand up straight and avoid any slouching. Make sure your elbows are locked out in front of you by sliding your hands down the two belt straps. Look inside (to the right) of your left leg rather than at your knee if you're having problems focusing.

Modified Stakes

1: When you twist, your abdominal muscles on one side battle against the back muscles on the other, which is where the benefits and the mechanics of the action reside. However, even if your feet are hip-width apart, some postures might cause your belly button to move forward or backward in respect to your neck. The radial pressures exerted during a twist improve both spinal mobility and strength. Hip and minor facet arthritis, back pain, musculoskeletal disorders, and a lack of core strength are among conditions that may benefit from them.

2: Patients with ankylosing spondylitis, severe scoliosis, a recent colostomy, a history of complete hip replacement (posterior approach), or a history of shoulder dislocation or shoulder replacement are not excellent candidates.

3: Moving on to the Third Stage, Marichyasana

4: You should switch places in your seat.

This position has a number of health benefits, and its mechanism of action is well established, since the vagus nerve travels via the neck, rib cage, and its contents (the lungs and big blood arteries), the stomach, and (to a lesser extent) the lumbar region. The vagus nerve is the longest nerve in the body, and research suggests it might help control hunger due to its proximity to the reward centres of the brain. Technically speaking, this posture mechanically extends the linings of the oesophagus, stomach, and duodenum.

If you have had a recent herniated disc, severe scoliosis, spinal fixation through Harrington rod, Cotrel-Dubousset, or fusion procedures, ankylosing spondylitis, or have had any of these disorders in the past, you should not get a tattoo (for example, after shoulder or hip replacement or due to severe arthritis).

Recommendations:

Straighten your spine as you take a deep breath in, and maintain that posture while you twist your body more on the exhale. A blanket may be used to support your lower body for optimal comfort. One should begin at the bottom rib and gradually move up to the more difficult variant of the stance. This prevents over-tightening of the muscles that line the inside of the thoracic cage.

Chapter: 8

Staying Safe to Gain the Benefits

HOW TO AVOID GETTING HURT

Even if you're practising yoga to help you lose weight, it's vital to understand that there are a lot of circumstances beyond your control that could limit your success. Sir Isaac Newton's first law asserts that for every action, there is an equal and opposite reaction. Don't we also generally expect consequences from anything that acts? When it comes to weight-loss drugs, it seems like an understatement, considering that there are apparently five to ten bad side effects for every beneficial one. There are some possible negative side effects of yoga, but they are infrequent, modest, and controllable.

For study I co-wrote with Ellen Saltonstall and Susan Genis, we interviewed 33,000 yoga instructors and practitioners about their past with yoga-related injuries.

1: There were initially the apparent truths, such as how placing too much weight on one's head may lead to neck discomfort, or how bending forward for too long might lead to stiff hamstrings the following day. But the wider image, or overall impression, was a little startling. It was commonly understood that these three variables accounted for the great majority of unintentional injuries. We were taken aback when a second, unaffiliated investigation in Australia verified our findings.

2: Two key causes of yoga injuries are demonstrated by data from about 50,000 practitioners in two studies.

BEING OVERACTIVE:

Whether out of pride, arrogance, a drive for perfection, or an overzealous embrace of yoga, the major cause of even minor injury is striving to accomplish things that are now beyond your capabilities. This is how instructors who aspire to be "role models" for their kids get themselves into trouble. Yet a number of paradoxical outcomes from both the Australian study and our own research indicate the concept to be valid.

The urge to embody the platonic ideal and the general drive for perfection surpass common sense, resulting to more injuries among instructors than among their learners.

- Injuries are more prevalent in the classroom than when students are practising on their own, indicating a competitive and egocentric incentive for classroom activities.
- Injuries are more prevalent in males than in women. In schools where female students make up the majority, the idea is deployed slightly differently: males take notice of women, who are frequently more flexible and skilled, and pit their stronger muscles against their shorter range of motion, resulting in injury.

The remedy is to slow down. Know your limitations, and if you're unclear what they are, maintain a safe distance away from them. I like to think of an example where a person is walking through a desert with a pyramid and a palm tree in the distance that are both framed by the horizon. At some point during his voyage, he will pass by the palm tree and, later, the pyramid. He will, however, never go above the horizon. I mean, why not? Considering that with each step he takes, he will pull the horizon further away. If he continues travelling, however, he will ultimately reach a spot in the sand that represents the original horizon. In light of your yoga objectives and where you are at the time, that is as it should be. In your yoga practise, it's better to begin with realistic aims, and then work your way up to longer-term, more aspirational goals as your talents and confidence increase. At some time, you will be able to carry out tasks that, at first, would have placed you at danger of greater damage. However, there will still be some constraints, so be careful.

Different Alignment

Justify your usage of the term "alignment" here. Naturally curved spines and vital laxity in the joints of the limbs, notably the hips, knees, and shoulders, must be taken into consideration. Of fact, being overweight may make improper alignment worse, just as it might "naturally" occur in persons who are only striving to reduce two pounds. Some individuals overestimate their physical talents because of their stature, while others don't know what their muscles and joints should be able to perform. Unawareness of anatomy is frequent. After discussing this with a colleague, we decided to ask all of the novices in our yoga class to point out their livers. Half of the participants in the group placed their hands on their left sides. They require both direction and physiological awareness, both of which are strengthened with yoga practises.

By the time we're in our teens, we know just how much power we have over our bodies and how far we can push them. We sometimes do things that we should know better than to do because we want to push beyond our boundaries, whether it's via the desire for perfection, enthusiastic excitement, competitiveness, or just plain showing off. You can only practise a certain range of poses in the yoga I'm teaching you, and my recommendations are always within that range. Your physical talents and restrictions are intimately known only to you.

Safe yoga poses take into mind the amount of weight and force that your shoulders, hips, and knees can safely handle. Thus, the front thigh, shin, and foot are all in the same plane in Virabhadrasana I, the Warrior I. If not, the unstable knee, the hip, and the ankle will all be at danger from the uneven forces. Keep in mind that I propose milder and more safe approaches for introducing postures initially, as well as typical faults to avoid. If you're not sure what to do, don't.

INADEQUATE INSTRUCTION

This is the third most prevalent cause of injury while practising yoga. Which course should I join in? I rigorously adhere to the requirement that there must be one instructor or awake assistance for every fifteen children, or 10 at the very maximum. Ignoring new kids is the worst thing a teacher can do, as faulty habits are hard to overcome and may have deadly effects later on. Taking the wrong moves repeatedly may have unforeseen repercussions in yoga. The ratio of instructors to pupils is straightforward to calculate and use as a standard for new teachers.

However, there are additional elements of education that effect harm. Five years of classroom experience is recommended for any educator who would be working with a new student who has a special need, such as obesity. After that period of time, a teacher should have encountered enough instances of typical difficulties to know how to appropriately manage them. Your medical history and your aims for practising yoga should be disclosed with the instructor. The classroom should be pristine, bright, and spacious enough for the children to spread out and feel independent.

The following are some of the less evident aspects of the teacher-student relationship: Do you respect the teacher, have trust in what they are directing you to do, and feel at comfortable doing it? Is he or she more to your liking? Deciding on these topics may take several meetings, but you shouldn't feel trapped once you do. You may injure your body, but far more detrimentally, you might harm your enthusiasm. Stay on your set route at all costs.

PROSPEROUS ENDING

5'3 "I was **6** feet tall and **179** pounds. Adrienne As a student, you owe it to yourself to take advantage of the free promotion being offered by that yoga studio. She bought a pair of baggy shorts and a top at a discount after finishing her final examinations, and wore them straight from the shop to the studio. Her first reaction to yoga was lukewarm. After the **90**-minute course, she was exhausted, but she had such a fantastic time that she signed up for another 10 lessons before she left. She found herself adjusting her calendar to fit her yoga schedule, despite having only attended a single session and having plenty of time to adjust for other class hours. Fortunately, she managed to cram in all of the required classes and still had time to go to and from her yoga sessions. It was something of which I was completely ignorant. The girl sitting next to me in American history class said that she had noticed I had lost weight. The number on the scale had dropped from **179 to 165** when I weighed myself. The third week of school was when it happened.

Adrienne was a top student and accomplished yogi. She continued to practise yoga for an hour twice a week and now does a 20-minute session in her room every day. Just before Easter, she had another scale reading. She visits California over spring break and brings her yoga mat back to Michigan.

I really didn't give any thought to my weight. I really thought I was going to miss yoga. Regrettably, I haven't been frequenting any of Grand Rapids' numerous yoga studios, so I was blissfully unaware of the city's plethora of such institutions. Two 45-minute sessions a day helped me retain the stuff I had been studying at home. What my parents prepared for me for lunch and supper surprised me since I didn't like for it or consume as much of it as I used to.

I reasoned that if I did yoga first thing in the morning, it would make me very hungry. However, the inverse was in fact true. My mother said that she had never seen me being so wasteful with my meals

before. By the time finals came around, I weighed in the low 140s and was anticipating three A's and a B+. Although I made no special efforts toward each objective, I met both in little over four months. My longest exercise streak was two weeks. Because yoga has helped me so much in many areas of my life, I believe this to be the case.

For the last sixteen years, Adrienne has spent part of her week at a law firm in the Midwest. She weighs just 124 pounds despite being a mother of two and a regular at office celebrations. Both of her children, ages 5 and 9, practise yoga with her on a daily basis. What Adrienne has gone through is not unprecedented. It's further evidence that yoga may influence your state of mind and hunger levels even if you don't want for it to. She may have improved her grades independently of her weight loss by being more disciplined. Potentially, mitochondria are at play here. Before she began doing yoga, she wasn't particularly interested in any of these things, but that quickly changed.

Not everyone, however, has the same degree of emotional instability as Adrienne. She dabbled with yoga at first, but after realising its advantages, she became a dedicated practitioner. Some people may be more motivated to stick with a programme or effort if they have specific goals in mind. Yoga is a fantastic technique to develop your willpower, self-discipline, or whatever term you want. Doing yoga may help you concentrate better. Of course, that's not all it can do. One's appetite, food desires, and calorie consumption might all be influenced by this. The practise of yoga has the potential to alter a person's worldview, including their view of themselves and their connections to others.

Eating and digestion are "insidiously" redirected attention away from while you practise yoga. You often find yourself questioning whether your motives were logical, selfless, or self-serving after taking any kind of action. Your perspective will change as you become more aware of your body and mind, just as Adrienne's did when she informed me she now appreciates everything, including herself, more highly after practising yoga.

Yoga has been widely regarded as a path to enlightenment by writers for over 2,000 years. It is widely believed that yoga may improve not only your health and longevity, but also the quality of your experiences while you are still alive. This may be measured consciously, as with your weight, or subconsciously, as when your mitochondria and telomeres cooperate to preserve your health without you seeing it.

Chapter: 9

How to Design and Use Pose Sequences

Twelve specific yoga postures have been identified as aiding in weight loss. Is there a better way to put them to use so that we can reach our objectives? The question "which positions can you use, and when?" will help you assess your situation more accurately. We can do whatever we want in the hour or so before dinnertime these days.

TRANSFORMABLE COMPONENTS

The lack of a comfortable place to sit or lie down means that yoga can be practised anywhere, including at the office, in a meeting, at a game, on public transportation, and in many other settings. The need to be motionless for relatively short intervals cannot be discounted. Some excellent choices include the Mountain Pose (Tadasana), the Tree Pose (Vriksasana), the Warrior Pose (Virabhadrasana I), and the Twisted Triangle Pose (Parivrtta Trikonasana) (not when pregnant). The other three poses each have at least two variations, but Tadasana is the only one that remains constant. There are seven distinct capabilities combined into one. Seven minutes if you hold each for a full minute.

Constantly holding someone back

The seated postures and twists are crucial if you suffer from knee or ankle pain, spinal stenosis, plantar fasciitis, a spinal compression fracture, have trouble keeping your balance, or are travelling by car, plane, or train with a low ceiling.

The Camel Squat (**Ustrasana**), the Half Lord of the Fishes Squat (**Adho Mukha Svanasana**), and the Seated Twist (**Marichyasana III**; not suggested during pregnancy) are all safe and effective poses that pregnant women can do (**Ardha Matsyendrasana**; not recommended during pregnancy). If you're writing an important message over lunch and can't resist snacking on **french fries**, try kneeling in the backseat of your car or spinning in your chair.

Back problems are common, and they can be made worse by obesity, which can be very unpleasant for some people. People with spinal stenosis frequently practise the following three forward bends in rapid succession; their Sanskrit names, Janu Sirsasana, Paschimottanasana, and Ardha Baddha Padma Janusirsasana, respectively, do not have direct English translations. Herniated disc sufferers can benefit from the back stretches and increased circulation that the Camel, Bridge, and Locust yoga positions provide. For those suffering from cauda equina, facet syndrome, or spinal stenosis, bending forward can be a welcome relief.

Fights against hunger

Two hours of fasting is recommended prior to a yoga practise. However, if you practise a particular sequence of poses, it may aid digestion. Some yoga

practitioners claim that practising a specific sequence of poses causes them to feel full more quickly. The most beneficial and effective sequences will take on a variety of shapes and sizes, depending on the nature of the situation and its outcomes.
Common ones include Tadasana, Salabhash, Janu Sirsasana, and Marichyasana. Tadasana, also known as the mountain pose, is a calming yoga posture in which the practitioner stands tall and strong. Salabhasana tones muscles that improve posture and breathing mechanics and boosts energy, and it has been shown to reduce hunger by stimulating gastrointestinal stretch receptors. Janu Sirsasana stretches the same muscle tissue that was contracted in Salabhasana, stimulating the stretch receptors in the digestive organs. Legs, back, chest, and even the face are all relaxed in Marichyasana, which is meant to counteract the heightened condition brought on by Salabhasana. The stimulation of all three sections of the gastrointestinal system aids in appetite suppression and relaxation by releasing tension in the abdominal and chest areas. Following that sequence should leave you less hungry and with a more alert and peaceful disposition following practise. It's possible that only some of these functions are essential to your success. But it's vital to keep boredom from setting in and making you lose interest in the same physical exercise over and over again. Introducing more diversity into one's diet may lead to better appetite regulation and a more acute awareness of

one's own requirements. You should start using them without delay, as suggested by me. The more practise you have, the more likely you are to be able to create your own rules.

The Vriksasana and the Setu Bandha Sasana Make a Beautiful Couple.

Paschimottanasana

A Refreshing New Variety of Marichyasana and Ardha Combinations Virabhadrasana Janusirsasana Padma Baddha. Salabhasana translates to "Quiet Pose" in Sanskrit. As I strike Ardha Matsyendrasana, I fuse the Mountain Pose (Tadasana) with the Warrior stance (Ustrasana). Parivrtta Trikonasana is a balancing pose in which the practitioner raises all three horns in the air. Though all four of these sets may be done on any given day, most individuals simply do the first three on a regular basis (morning, afternoon, and night). You don't have to do one task from each set every day for four weeks since there are four sets; this allows for flexibility in the schedule to accommodate for things like job, travel, and other commitments. By learning and doing these routines, one may learn to manage, enhance, or otherwise change his or her emotional state.

If the idea of beginning something as foreign and unfamiliar as yoga is intimidating, try practising before only one meal every day to ease into it. For the next two weeks, do one of these sets 15-30 minutes before eating at the time of day when you plan to consume the maximum calories. That will first get you ready for what's coming, and second, it will teach you to respect the holiness of your body and the miracle of being alive. You'll probably have a better understanding of the influence that food has on your mood, sense of identity, and willingness to put up effort in almost any endeavour. You may find that you lose weight gradually.

Some very accomplished and flexible yogis could benefit from reducing some weight, despite the fact that yoga and being overweight are often at different extremities of the physical fitness continuum. After much deliberation, I have put up a brief sequence of "extra credit" asanas that dedicated yogis may do before chowing down.

“EXTRA CREDIT” POSES FOR EXPERIENCED YOGIS

There may be some yogis who have been overweight for years despite their practise, but it is unusual to encounter a yogi who is also overweight. Between fifteen and thirty minutes before to meals, all the positions we've specified will have been done, and some of them may have been done on purpose. If you aren't convinced by my previous points, maybe the ones below will convince you. Even seasoned yogis may struggle to perfect all of these positions. Before attempting any of the positions, make sure you have read the whole section dedicated to them. Following the description of the standard posture comes that of the "beginning" variation. It will provide those who have never worked before a far clearer picture of their future career paths.

Few of the really exceptional yogis I've met have ever attempted a headstand. Many people stay away from it since they have heard horror stories about how badly it may affect them. The victim's slouched position likely contributed to the severity of their injuries. Several Iyengar instructors and I have spent up to thirty minutes on our heads without any discomfort over the period of several decades. Often called the "**king of asanas**," this position deserves respect. The following guidelines are provided as a starting point; however, if you still have questions after reading them, it may be best to hire an instructor for your first attempts.

Its usefulness and functionality: Light on Yoga, written by **B.K.S. Iyengar**, is a bestseller for good reason; in the book's end, the author compiles a list of medical conditions and the asana that can alleviate their symptoms. Three-quarters of the asanas we recommend begin in headstand (**Sirsasana**). The headstand is often disregarded in Western yoga due to safety concerns about neck injuries, glaucoma, and cerebrovascular illnesses, as well as concerns about bigger, potentially more litigious yoga classes.

Even if you don't suffer from any of the aforementioned ailments, using **hCG** to reprogram your digestive and circulatory systems is an excellent approach to get insight into your body and how it works.

When breathing while upside down, the diaphragm has the additional task of supporting the body's heaviest organs—the stomach and intestines. This trains your respiratory muscles to work harder and forces you to breathe more deliberately.

Heart conditions such as congestive failure and abnormal heart rhythms Wolff-Parkinson-White syndrome, severe hyper-or hypotension, glenohumoral (shoulder) dislocation, Sprengel's deformity, wide-angle and narrow-angle glaucoma, fracture, muscle imbalance, vascular accident (stroke), vascular disease, cerebral or carotid aneurism, epidural or subdural hematoma, and traumatic brain injury (TBI) Possible Helpful Hints: Do something with the attentional centre of your mind. Don't lean on your forehead or the back of your head if you need to keep your balance. The fontanelles, which are bony projections at the top of the skull, should bear the bulk of the pressure. Even seasoned yogis will need to make many changes to their arms and the posture of their heads during Sirsasana to accommodate their bodies' natural ebb and flow. In order to prevent kyphosis, lordosis, and swayback, it's best to keep your spine in a neutral position.

The "king of postures" is frequently omitted from even teacher training courses and yoga seminars, so here is some good advice for first-timers. My friends and I who share my hobbies have found that when performed correctly, headstands seldom cause any kind of injury.

THROUGH THE POSE

1: A blanket may be folded in half and used as a room divider.

2: Put your palms together and interlace your fingers fully.
3: Squat down so that your forearms create a right triangle in the centre of the blanket.
4: The fourth step is to place the apex of the triangle just over your fontanelles. Stretch your arms behind your back until you can reach up and touch your own head.
5: When going in on tiptoe into your eyes, keep your feet symmetrical so that you may distribute your weight more evenly between your forearms and your thighs. The risk of injury increases the more you stretch your elbows.
6: Sirsasana is the first yoga pose, and on the sixth inhalation, you should begin to straighten your body by lifting your feet off the ground. You may have to bend your knees slightly at first, but with some practise you should be able to execute it with perfectly straight legs.
So that your legs don't droop, it's vital to have some range of motion in your hips. If you draw a line from your ankles to your hips to your shoulders and then up to your ears, you'll have a decent body form.
Roll your shoulders up and back, down and away from your ears while you take a few deep breaths. Do not move your arms from their current positions.
"Takeoff Pose" (**Sirsasana**) is a common name for a yoga posture that many people refer to as "Sirsasana." Sirsasana, sometimes called "Legs-Up-The-Stand." Sirsasana, often known as the "almost there" position,

Sirsasana

Change which forearm is carrying the weight, and move the weight back and forth between your elbows and wrists. The goal is to be able to hold the position for five minutes and fifty seconds. To complete releasing the headstand, Step 11 must be done backwards. Get on your knees, but be ready to spring up to your toes as soon as you touch down. Use both legs at once for the ascent and the downhill, as challenging as it may seem at first.

As an Introduction for the Novices

(Remember, you're going to need a spotter standing behind you so you don't completely wipe out.)

1: Place the blanket against the wall and sit with your back against it, legs extended out in front of you until your feet contact the wall.

2: Identify your position on the chair.

3: The next step is to roll onto your back while kneeling in the appropriate place.

4: The fourth gesture is a reverse hand clasp.

5: Position yourself with your back against the wall, hands on the blanket so that your little fingers create a right triangle, and your head in the middle of the triangle.

6: You may extend your legs out by propping your feet up on the wall at a shallow angle (step 6). Everything above the waist line should be almost vertical.

7: Sirsasana, the abbreviated version, may be utilised to locate this specific area. Supported by the wall (easier version). Try at least 30 seconds, then increase if necessary.

8: Go down the wall until you reach Step 8. Before getting down on your hands and knees, check that both of your feet are touching the floor.

9: If you lose your balance and start to fall backward, release whatever objects you're hanging on to and bend your knees to cushion the fall as much as possible. Fears about falling behind are unfounded.

10: It's time to set up the blanket in the corner of a room with the aid of a buddy once you've gotten the hang of it and practised a few times.

The **second method**, which is more difficult for beginners, is inverting oneself in a corner of a room such that your outside ankles or heels touch the perpendicular walls. Practicing against a single wall causes the body to adopt an arch, which causes the legs to collapse and the stomach to protrude. That's bad for the sensory systems in your brain and might give you a headache or neck pain.

1: A blanket should be tucked into a secret spot.

2: Bring the corner of the blanket that you've folded in half between your knees.

3: To a full headstand as instructed, using assistance from a buddy if necessary.

4: Raise your feet up on the wall in the corner.

Step forward and in toward the centre until your feet are no longer touching the walls. The completion of this task may need many, extended meetings. If the outside world gets too dangerous, you should take refuge behind the fort's walls. In **7 minutes and 30**

seconds, you will be able to stand for **5 minutes and 30 seconds** if you begin by standing for **30 seconds**. Do the whole headstand with a buddy looking on, if at all possible. Maybe being alone for another week or two may help you regain your sanity.

Pose with a twist, also known **as Parivrtta Parsvakonasana**

Uses and benefits: This is as twisted as a posture can get. The shin of one leg firmly planted on the floor and the forearm of the opposing arm attempting to rotate your body provide tremendous leverage. Torque will be applied at full capacity to any unrestrained portion of the digestive system. Due to their position at the centre of the body's torque, the oesophagus, stomach, and duodenum are subjected to the most stretching. This position is ideal for those suffering with piriformis syndrome, a type of sciatica, since it stretches the piriformis muscle while simultaneously engaging the primary muscle groups above and below it. This pose may be among the group of twelve that can reverse osteoporosis because it applies a lot of torque to the vertebral bodies and puts the front and back hips under different but equal pressure, both of which lead to increased bone deposition.

Total hip replacement (posterior approach), severe knee or hip arthritis, anterior cruciate or medial meniscal tear, colostomy, and pregnancy are all absolute contraindications.

THROUGH THE POSE

1: Spread your feet about 4.5 metres (about 5 feet) apart.
2: Step out ninety degrees with your right foot, then step in thirty degrees with your left.
3: In a standing position, bend your right knee to 90 degrees so that your right shin is perpendicular to the floor and your right thigh is horizontal.
4: Spread your right foot's weight out to its individual toes.
5: With one fluid motion, rotate your upper body to the right, bringing your left hip, chest, and shoulder forward, and curling the outside of your left armpit around the outside of your right knee.
6: Your right arm should be at a 45-degree angle behind your ear and over your head, while your left palm will be next to your right foot.
7: Join your twisted left leg and right arm to your twisted upper body to form a single diagonal line.
8: To prevent your right chest from protruding upward, reach from the outside of your left foot and your heel to your right fingers, and pull back on the mat with your left hand.
9: Take even, relaxed breaths.
10: Maintain the position for a full 30 seconds.

A variant with less difficulty

1: Stand with your back against a wall, a few inches away, and your feet four and a half to five feet apart.
2: With your left foot, pivot it so it's parallel to the wall; with your right foot, pivot it inward 30 degrees.

3: Keep your upper body upright as you bend your left knee to 90 degrees, bringing your left shin in line with your upper thigh.
4: Centre 50 percent of your bodyweight over the left foot's four corners. Your right foot is responsible for the other half.
5: Kneel on the mat by bending your right knee.
6: Position your right elbow slightly beyond your left knee and in touch with the outside of your left thigh; place your right and left hands on the wall; and drive your right hip, chest, and shoulder forward and to the left.
7: Keep your left shin upright while using your right hand for balance and twisting, and use your left hand on the wall for stability and more rotation.
8: Turn not only at the shoulders but also at the narrowest part of your waist, in the space between your ribs and your low back.
9: If your right elbow is touching your left thigh, you may prevent your chest from protruding forward by pulling the elbow (without really moving it) toward your upper leg and torso (not pictured).
10: Keep your breathing regular and relaxed.
11: Hold the position for 30 seconds.

Urdhva Dhanurasana: The Reversed Shoulder-Breaker Pose

The Wheel

This difficult stance causes an excessive arch, which pushes the digestive system to its limits. The biliary tract, which runs from the liver to the gall bladder and eventually connects with a tube from the pancreas, is probably also stretched. Both the ovaries and fallopian tubes lengthen, as does the bladder, ureters, and urethra. You can probably suppress your hunger by extending from your throat to your ankles.

This pose, by elongating and arching the back, mimics a key movement in physical therapy based on the work of McKenzie, which is effective for herniated discs. This movement involves creating a partial vacuum at the front of the intervertebral spaces between the vertebral bodies, which pulls the disc material toward its proper location, away from the nerve roots emerging from the back of the spinal column.

All those who suffer from osteopenia or osteoporosis may benefit from this posture because of the enormous arch it places on the back, which in turn stimulates the spinal discs to produce more bone mineral density.

Last but not least, in this energising position, a negative view is next to impossible to sustain. Even while there is no way to ensure that your mood will "permanently" improve, even a short period of respite might make you feel better. Sacroiliac joint derangement, spinal stenosis, facet syndrome, anterolisthesis, spondylolysis, Klippel-Feil syndrome, Sprengel's deformity, and cerebrovascular illness are all conditions that should not be treated with this method.

THROUGH THE POSE

1: Lay flat on your back on a sticky mat.

2: Stand with your feet parallel and hip-width apart, and your knees bent.
3: With palms down and fingers angled slightly outward, dig your hands into the mat beneath your shoulders.
4: Put your hands down on the mat and push your fingers into the ground while you bring your shoulder blades down toward your hips.
5: Take a deep breath in and arch your back ribs gently from head to toe as you stretch your spine, raise your pelvis, and lift your shoulders off the ground.
6: Using just your head, hands, and feet on the mat, regain your equilibrium and sense of direction.
7: Pay close attention to the soles of both feet.
8: Use your hands to exert enough pressure on the mat so your chest rises high enough to rest the crown of your head on the floor.
9: Relax and take a few deep breaths.
10: As you start to climb, take a deep breath in and hold it until your elbows are absolutely straight.
11: Feet and palms on the floor, stop again for another deep, calm breath.
12: Now, without moving your feet, push them into the mat in a direction away from your head and body. This will lift and advance your chest, putting your sternum further over your chin and your shoulders precisely over your hands.
13: Take a few deep, pleasant breaths at your highest point, with your arms outstretched, hollow under your armpits, shoulder blades and back ribs

propelling your chest forward, and your head hung above your spinal column.

14: Descend gently by releasing the backward pressure on your feet, the downward push of the hands and elbows, and the backward thrust of the shoulders. As you gradually bend your elbows, this happens. Focus on making this a cohesive effort.

15: Let the back of your head rest on the mat for a few breaths before continuing on.

16: Straightening the elbows helps to lift the body even further.

Benefits and how it works: Like more sedate forward bends, this strenuous position will compress stomach contents. Unlike most others, it will also aggressively recruit abdomen and back muscles to function in synchronous synchronisation as front-to-back balance is key to the position. The stance is thrilling and takes your thoughts, your emotions, and, in my experience, even your metabolism away from a focus on eating.

Like Trianga Mukhaikapada Paschimottanasana, this posture accentuates the alternating and reciprocal motions of the ankles. By reversing the pathological co-contraction of ankle flexors and extensors, the primary source of fascia-tearing pressures on the arches of the feet, this is helpful for patients with plantar fasciitis.

Contraindications: (Unquestionably): posterior hip replacement;Abdominal or inguinal hernia, severe osteoporosis, a severe or recent herniated disc, knee pathology such as meniscal or cruciate ligamentous rips, severe knee or hip arthritis or knee replacement, sprained ankle

Helpful hints: Manually pull the bent leg's calf muscles to the sides to allow you to sit on both ischial bones. Maintain an upright posture. It's your foot that should be brought to your head, not

THROUGH THE POSE

1: Sit on the inside of your left calf with your left knee bent under you and your right leg extended straight out in front of you. If you lean in any direction, it will be to the right. Equalize the weight on your sit bones to address this. If support is needed for the right buttock, use a block or blanket there.

2: Bend and elevate your right knee. Either grasp your left wrist with your right hand or hold your right foot with both hands.

3: Exhale as you straighten your right leg and elevate it to your forehead or, better yet, your chin.

4: Use your arms to bring your head up in line with your vertical leg and toward your foot.

5: While breathing normally for 30 seconds, gradually rise higher with each exhale.

6: Slowly drop your right leg as you inhale and exhale.

7: Do the same thing on the other side.

Less demanding variants

1: Balance might be a concern in this stance. If so, sit with your heel against a wall for front-to-back support and both hands on the mat to avoid falling to the back.

2: Loop a belt immediately under the ball of the straight or nearly straight leg. Hold the belt while you elevate the leg toward the vertical. While doing so, rest the free hand on the ground or a block at the bent leg's foot.

KNOWING WHEN TO SAY WHEN

A ABILITY TO READ CLOCKS Martha, my cousin, spent a week with us at the lake house in Connecticut. She lamented her aching feet every afternoon. On a few occasions, however, her fear kept her from joining us as we walked along the beach at night. She was a phenomenal clinical psychologist and school administrator. Small, she stood only 5 feet tall and weighed only 160 pounds.

After carefully examining her feet, I didn't notice anything out of the ordinary that would necessitate an X-ray. There is no discomfort in wearing these shoes.

We're at a complete loss for words. She addressed the question with a pleasant tone and an enticing grin on her face.

A hasty and thoughtless response was mine. As soon while I saw him, I exclaimed, "You know, as your arms and chest and legs get gigantic, your feet don't shift. They don't vary much from one year to the next. Martha said she had been gazing at her feet for a moment. In a significant way, "quite a bit."

The issue arises when one's feet don't keep pace with the rest of one's body in terms of growth.

"Right." This is a sign of increasing pressure in the same region."True." Asked about their hiking experience, "Have you ever gone hiking with a backpack?" One of my all-time favourite: Did the discomfort in your feet persuade you to stop? In fact, I find myself agreeing with you. That's all. You may put away your other bag.

Upon comprehending her impotence, Martha, aged 49, looked up and exclaimed, "So what can I do?" Just what is in those terrible drugs, anyway? Negatively enjoyable physical exercise is the worst. Consider yourself really lucky if your wife is a competent chef. If you need me, I won't be available throughout my trip.

I promised her she could stop eating sooner than usual if she ate whenever she wanted. Since the stomach, like the bladder, is made up of smooth muscles, it can stretch to accommodate almost any form of food. Your stomach could become smaller if you fast for a week or longer, eating just 5% of what you usually consume.

Well, I guess I'll simply go hungry for a week." Laughingly, Martha retorted. I would have said one hour if pushed. Do you recall that it was a no-no to snack on cookies after 4 o'clock when you were a kid?

They warned us that if we did this, supper at 5:30 p.m. would be impossible.

Ingesting the cookies, having their sugars metabolised, and then having glucose circulated through our veins and capillaries shut off the developing hunger centres in our brains. The same thing will happen if you leave the table at 7:30 and are still hungry.

I could see she was starting to get what I was saying, so I argued that "dinner is digested and very fast turns off the hunger areas in our adult brains."
You could have been hungry when you left supper, but by nine o'clock, you won't be. This is true even if you haven't eaten since 7:30 am. Before then, my hunger level had dropped to 5%.
Martha stuck to this plan and dropped weight steadily at a rate of around a pound per week for quite some time. Down April, she was happy to report that she had settled in at her target weight of 140. In a sense, her return the following summer was like a "before and after" advertisement. She seemed healthy, content, and typical.
When appropriate, I use tenets of yoga's guiding philosophy and method into my clinical work. My method with my family member was not yoga, but it was helpful nevertheless. Patients whose excess weight was a clear contributing cause of the onset of their back pain were my first priority while treating conditions like herniated discs and dislocated sacroiliac joints. Many people's lives have been altered significantly because of it.
Not getting enough rest and stuffing oneself silly
The information loop between the stomach and the brain isn't always correct. The second time-dependent mechanism by which yoga reduces hunger is through the activation of stretch receptors in the stomach, which in turn suppresses activity in the brain's hunger-inducing centres. As I said before, this pattern explains why the feedback loop is at its

most powerful around noon and just a fraction as effective after midnight. Anyone worried about their weight should avoid eating at night since it greatly increases their chance of acquiring weight. Those who can't sleep are usually found in the kitchen, finishing up the last of the leftovers or an entire carton of ice cream.

If you can't sleep and have to wake up to grab food from the fridge at 3 a.m., try some yoga. The stretch receptors in your oesophagus, stomach, and duodenum are less responsive after midnight, so you should avoid eating at that time. It's less likely that you'll hurt yourself if you know how to put yourself to sleep.

If you wake up in the middle of the night and can't get back to sleep, try doing seven minutes of yoga in bed.

This notice arrived about a week before the deadline for me to submit the book to the publisher. Pardon I'm sorry, Loren; I spoke too soon.

I tried out your new leg stretch, but I made several breathing mistakes and ended myself sleeping for four hours. Put simply, I got rid of the tranquillizers. Please know how much I value your help.

This complete yoga routine may be performed while lying in bed. I've seen positive responses from patients using this method in my clinic. It may take some practise, but good sleep will eventually become second nature. Regrettably, many readers nod off long before the last page is turned. To put things in perspective, I would say that you have a

90% chance of success. It is divided into three sections. All participants begin in a prone position:

PART 1

The very first yoga position is the Supta Padangusthasana.

(There is no good English equivalent.)

It's comforting to know that your snoring won't wake anybody up. In addition to helping persons with osteoporosis stretch their hamstrings without putting unnecessary pressure on their spines, this position has the potential to promote relaxation and better sleep. Hamstring stretch receptors communicate with the calming centres of the brain (the cortex and the basal ganglia).

Some injuries prevent patients from undergoing this operation, including idiopathic sacroiliac joint syndrome, a torn hamstring, or an adductor tear. Those who have been diagnosed with sleep apnea should undergo regular monitoring following the initial diagnosis. Some patients with gastroesophageal reflux disease (GERD) find relief by placing a bolster under their chest and head, although this is not recommended for those with severe upper respiratory infections such as asthma attacks or bronchitis flare-ups.

If you find that sleeping with a belt helps, don't take it off until morning. Keep your elbows as straight as possible by holding the belt with both hands and pulling it up with your hands. After extending fully with straight elbows, pull down on your shoulders to bring them back to the bed.

CONFIDENCE IN ONE'S POSITION

1: Extend your legs behind you and lie flat on your back. You may forego the pillow.

2: Rest the back of your right knee on the bed, and raise your left thigh until your left knee is bent and your leg is vertical.

3: The third step is to raise the left foot off the ground and support it with one or two hands. This may be done by gripping the big toe with the first and second fingers of the left hand, or by holding both ends of a belt that wraps around the foot just behind the ball of the foot.

4: Reach over with your left hand and grab the right wrist, or slide your fingers as high up the belt as they will go.

5: Keep your elbows straight and your shoulders lifted slightly off the bed as you extend your arms as far as you feel comfortable doing so. Bring your left knee closer to your forehead as you inhale and tense your quads.

6: The sixth instruction is to retighten the quadriceps to keep the leg in a rigid position.

7: Keep this position for 30 seconds before switching legs.

The first version is the most straightforward.

If your left leg is not yet at a correct angle, practise this position by bending your right leg and placing your foot level on the bed (90 degrees). It's possible that stretching your hamstrings in this way can help you straighten your left leg. It may be easier to extend your left leg while maintaining a stable pelvis if you lean backward from the hips.

The second step is to maintain your right knee bent as you slide your foot outside and then extend your leg at the heel to bring your right foot forward.

Third, whether sitting or standing, you must apply pressure to the upper sacrum in order to tilt the pelvis and extend the hamstrings.

For the left leg, the major action is an outward push since the belt pulls the left foot in (which maintains the arch in the lower back). The lower back will twist clockwise when the left leg or foot is brought toward the head. Once you've found the most comfortable posture for yourself, take a moment to look around and let go of any tension you notice, focusing on your stomach, shoulders, neck, and face. Repeat the procedure on the other side. You'll be more prepared for whatever lies ahead after striking this stance, which promotes patience and perseverance.

Second Choice

To completely extend your knee if you still can't after raising your leg to a **60-degree angle**, hold the back of your left thigh with both hands and elevate your leg, maintaining your knee as straight as possible.

When one knee is bent to roughly fifty degrees, some people's hamstrings are so tight that they cannot bend their knee at all. There, the bone itself takes the brunt of the pressure, rather than the muscle. In such situation, you should hold the back of your thigh and draw your leg toward you. Maintain as much knee straightness as you can.

Part: 2

The First and Second Viloma

(No good English translation)

You may practise deep breathing with Viloma I or Viloma II. There are two parts to this activity, and they both have names. Hold still! Each one may *be* completed while laying flat.

What's in it for you, and how it works: It is my belief that this way of breathing dissects the pleura into its component layers, the visceral pleura and the parietal pleura, which cover each lung. Vagus nerve sensory fibres are densely packed inside these tissues. Their stimulation reduces the "fight or flight" reaction and increases the "rest and digest" response, all of which contribute to a more restful night's sleep.

Regular monitoring is necessary for patients with a sleep apnea diagnosis both before and throughout treatment. Those who suffer from gastroesophageal reflux disease may discover that placing a bolster under their chest improves their night's sleep. When you have a serious case of asthma, bronchitis, or an upper respiratory infection, you shouldn't take any chances.

An important piece of advise is to maintain a steady breathing rate throughout the three phases of inhalation described in the first section and the three phases of exhalation described in the second section.

IMAGINE THIS, JUST AS AN EXAMPLE:

1: Please be quiet for a minute. Since breathing in demands a lot of muscular effort, you may speed up the process by keeping your chest up as you do it.
2: Maintain an open chest while exhaling slowly and deeply via the nose.
3: After a brief pause to allow the exhaled air to settle, the third step is to inhale slowly and deeply for one-third of a full breath. When pausing again, rather of letting your tongue or neck hold you back, focus on keeping your diaphragm from falling into your chest.
4: Inhale deeply to take in the remaining two-thirds of the air once number four has taken a brief rest.
5: Cause another halt without suffocating.
6: After a few seconds, inhale the remaining air to fully fill your lungs.
7: When you feel your lungs becoming full, pause for a while and exhale softly.
8: Correct, take several deep breaths and calm yourself. The amount of blood that reaches the brain and lungs is impacted by the blood pressure in the chest. Restoring these intricate but crucial cycles calls for regular breathing.
9: Do it all over again, and then take a few deep breaths to unwind.
10: Repeat the procedure twice more, for a grand total of three times through.
11: After taking a regular breath, you should repeat the Viloma II.

A Second Viloma
(Soon To Follow)

1: Take a few deep breaths in and then exhale completely.
2: let out a casual third of the air that you just took in. It may be feasible to halt exhalation without moving the tongue or neck by blocking the diaphragm's upward movement.
3: Hold your breath for three seconds, and then let all the air out of your lungs at once.
4: Hold your breath for a second, then let it all out.
5: Resume a regular breathing pattern.
6: Each time you go through the three-step process of exhaling, you should take two extra deep breaths in between.

The first step in achieving restful sleep is mastering the art of breathing control. A few wild guesses are thrown in for good measure at the end. These meditative practises were developed by Kashmiri Shaivite Vairagya Tantric teachers. 3 They are designed to help people connect with their inner selves and the greater whole.

It's crucial to maintain a steady one-minute mental loop in which you cycle over the same nine ideas. Please don't let the clock distract you. The aim is to focus really hard on it until it gradually disappears from your mind. The next idea is ready whenever you are. You may need to go back to the original source the first few times you put the concepts into practise, but within a few days, you should be able to recall them on your own. You may see a summary of all nine recommendations below:

Love

Radiance
Unity
Health
Strength
Abundance
Wisdom
Light-as-air

Contrary to popular belief, outer space is not a secure location.

Patanjali, the founder of yoga, remarked, "Yoga decreases mental inconstancy," which he meant to mean through the act of routinely forcing oneself to sleep. This is beneficial to one's sense of self-worth and to genuine pleasure.

Chapter: 10

From the Practical to the Sublime

1: Anxiety and stress relief techniques like yoga and meditation

The thoughts in our heads are always in flux, moving from one time period to the next and back again. Constant mental and planning activity has physical and emotional costs. One's mind and body may be trained to cooperate via the various yoga practises. Yoga is an integrated practise that aims to lower stress and improve health via a variety of physical postures (asanas), breath work, and meditative reflection. Focus your whole concentration on the asanas. Philosopher Arthur Schopenhauer characterises this state, when one's anxieties and concerns evaporate and they become one with the universe, as the "joy from realisation of the observer's emptiness and oneness with Nature."

2: Set your spirit on fire.

Yoga is an inside journey, not merely a set of physical poses. Yoga has been shown to boost self-esteem, concentration, and appreciation of oneself in times of low mood. By stimulating the brain and inspiring it to make better decisions, yoga provides a solid framework within which to discover one's life's purpose and meaningful path. If you want to expand your awareness of your inner and outward capabilities, a yoga class or retreat led by a seasoned instructor is the way to go.

3: The Big Picture, So to Speak

It might be challenging to concentrate on your spiritual practise if you have a million and one other things to accomplish. They practise yoga to keep it all together, including a 9-to-5 job, a partner, and maybe even children. If you're a beginner to yoga, you may worry that you're not quite reaching that "sublime state," and that worry can show up in your practise. If you're having trouble making this connection, maybe you need to go on a yoga retreat. Spending time in nature, doing yoga, eating healthily, and getting enough of sleep can put you in a better position to undergo the type of metamorphosis that will enable you to live more sublimely once you return to your usual routine. If you are able to completely awaken and embrace your real nature while on your yoga retreat, the lessons you learn will have a deeper influence on your life.

4: Harmonize Yourself With Nature.
Yoga classes during retreats are often held in scenic outdoor settings. Is there any other way to escape the bustle of city life while yet spending time in nature and recharging one's own batteries? You may deepen your ties to nature and experience self-awareness in ways that are difficult or impossible to replicate at home. Therefore, cultivating such a connection with nature and the innermost aspects of yourself may lead to a sublime condition in which you love yourself and the people around you.

5: Be yourself in front of others.
Asanas (postures), mantras (sounds), meditative practises (stillness of mind), and a good attitude are all components of yoga. All of these problems are handled by the instructors. By learning more about yoga's history, anatomy, and purpose, you may enhance your practise and develop a stronger sense of self. After then, it's on you to reflect on your own capacity for the sublime and remain open to the kinds of experiences that "take[s] us beyond ourselves."
Wordsworth penned the following lines in his poem "Lines Composed a Few Miles Above Tintern Abbey" If you want to "look more magnificent," you need to be in a "good mood," where "the burden of the mystery, where the heavy and tired weight of all this unfathomable cosmos is alleviated."
6: Just how important is goal achievement to the goal regulation process?

It has been shown that giving people prizes on a regular basis makes them more productive. However, self-starting is required. It is generally agreed upon by experts that individuals have less willpower, or the ability to act on their own wishes instead of giving in to harmful impulses, throughout the day. You'll have greater control over yourself throughout the day if you get up and going early. Be kind with yourself every morning after a restful night's sleep. Taking periodic breaks throughout the day may help you maintain a strong willpower "muscle" and avoid its tiredness and weakness. Put aside a few minutes to focus only on your breathing as you shut your eyes.

Be fair to yourself and don't lock the fridge if you tend to open it at inconvenient times, like the middle of the day or the wee hours of the night. Put whatever it is you're considering swallowing in your mouth, give it a good chew, and see whether you're still interested in swallowing it after that. Perhaps what you need is really stored on the second shelf of the fridge, and you know just how to get there. Admitting you're hungry is quite OK, and may even be funny. Whatever the circumstance may be, it shouldn't be an excuse to give in.

When you have the want to consume something you know you will later regret, you have the power and the responsibility to make a different option. Saying to yourself, "I can't have the ice cream in the freezer because..." or "I'm choosing not to have the ice cream because..." is a certain way to guarantee that you'll end up eating it anyhow. You may act at your own discretion. According to David Seymour, who has coined the term "choice pandemic," obesity is mostly the result of individual decision-making. But there's another aspect of this reality that can't be ignored. It's up to the individual to make the decision to lose weight and keep it off if they are overweight. One and probably many others, have benefited by trying to put off pleasure for a little while. You can tell yourself, "Yes, I'll take what's left in that pint of chocolate ice cream that's in the freezer" to fulfil your want for something sweet. But I won't be able to give it justice right now. I have about 10 minutes to kill here. However, I could always put it off till the next day. If you don't remove it from the freezer immediately, I will throw it away. It is also suggested that you get rid of any temptations you may have at home.

I guess it's time to speak about objectives. Before starting a diet or exercise regimen to assist you lose weight, you need obviously make a plan. To achieve your goals, you should be as detailed as possible. Being imprecise decreases one's chances of success. Writing out your goals is a smart move. Their objectives might be thought of as either immediate or more far-reaching. In order to successfully reduce weight, you must do both.

You can get along just fine without a daily, weekly, or monthly schedule. However, keeping the weight off is also an important element of the plan. You are dooming yourself to disappointment if you don't fully dedicate yourself to the new ways of living you're trying out (such your diet, yoga practise, and bedtime). Choose something that will have far-reaching effects on your daily routine.

If you don't make a long-term commitment, your arrogance will grow dangerously. Extreme lifestyle adjustments, such as a lifetime abstinence from sugar, are possible for certain individuals. If you follow that approach, you may be able to lose weight and keep it off for at least a year or two. The problem is that it's easy to slip back into old routines. Now is the time to really benefit from yoga's many advantages.

I've said it before and I'll say it again: yoga's advantages aren't limited to the body. The spirituality and compassion of the author shine through in this piece. Your hunger will decrease and you will get a new outlook on life if you practise yoga consistently, even if just for a short period of time. Your perspective has changed. You could have a new perspective on the situation now. Your feelings towards food have changed. You now have a renewed appreciation for life and for yourself.

www.ingramcontent.com/pod-product-compliance
Lightning Source LLC
LaVergne TN
LVHW010605160826
845677LV00013B/3248

* 9 7 9 8 8 4 7 3 6 2 8 3 2 *